TIME

Your Body
A User's Guide

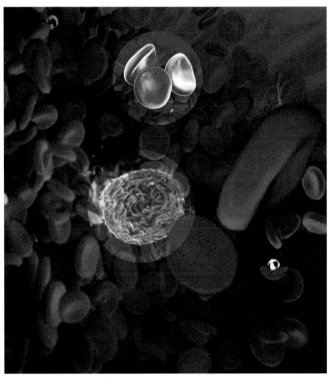

River of life *Elements of human blood include red blood cells (high-lighted at top), which carry oxygen from the lungs to body tissue; white blood cells (center), which attack intruders in the bloodstream; and tiny platelets (right), which help blood clot and thus stop bleeding. All float in a plasma solution*

TIME

MANAGING EDITOR Richard Stengel
DEPUTY MANAGING EDITOR Adi Ignatius
ART DIRECTOR Arthur Hochstein

Your Body: A User's Guide

SENIOR EDITOR Alice Park
EDITOR Kelly Knauer
DESIGNER Ellen Fanning
PICTURE EDITOR Patricia Cadley
WRITER/RESEARCHER Matthew McCann Fenton
COPY EDITOR Bruce Christopher Carr

LIAISON, ANATOMICAL TRAVELOGUE, INC: Atilla Ambrus

TIME INC. HOME ENTERTAINMENT
PUBLISHER Richard Fraiman
GENERAL MANAGER Steven Sandonato
EXECUTIVE DIRECTOR, MARKETING SERVICES Carol Pittard
DIRECTOR, RETAIL & SPECIAL SALES Tom Mifsud
DIRECTOR, NEW PRODUCT DEVELOPMENT Peter Harper
ASSISTANT DIRECTOR, NEWSSTAND MARKETING Laura Adam
ASSISTANT DIRECTOR, BRAND MARKETING Joy Butts
ASSOCIATE COUNSEL Helen Wan
SENIOR BRAND MANAGER, TWRS/M Holly Oakes
BOOK PRODUCTION MANAGER Suzanne Janso
DESIGN AND PREPRESS MANAGER Anne-Michelle Gallero
ASSISTANT BRAND MANAGER Michela Wilde

SPECIAL THANKS
Glenn Buonocore, Tymothy Byers, Susan Chodakiewicz, Margaret Hess,
Brynn Joyce, Robert Marasco, Brooke Reger, Mary Sarro-Waite,
Ilene Schreider, Adriana Tierno, Alex Voznesenskiy

This book features the writing, reporting and illustrations of many TIME staff members, including: William Lee Adams,
John Cloud, Dan Cray, Lisa Takeuchi Cullen, Nancy Gibbs, Christine Gorman, Sanjay Gupta, M.D., Eban Harrell, Kristen Kloberd,
Jeffrey Kluger, Betsy Kroll, Michael Lemonick, Joe Lertola, J. Madeiline Nash, Lori Oliwenstein, Alice Park, Carolyn Sayre,
Andrea Sachs, Elizabeth Salleme, Kate Stinchfield, Lon Tweeten, Claudia Wallis, Bryan Walsh, Daniel Williams

Copyright 2008 Time Inc. Home Entertainment
Published by TIME Books, Time Inc. • 1271 Avenue of the Americas New York, NY 10020

ISBN 10: 1-60320-050-9
ISBN 13: 978-1-60320-050-9
LOC: 2008907869

We welcome your comments and suggestions about TIME Books. Please write to us at: TIME Books • Attention: Book Editors • PO Box
11016 • Des Moines, IA 50336-1016

If you would like to order any of our hardcover Collector's Edition books, please call us at 1-800-327-6388 (Monday through Friday, 7
a.m.–8 p.m., or Saturday, 7 a.m.–6 p.m., Central time).

PRINTED IN THE UNITED STATES OF AMERICA

Editor's Note: Illuminating Visions

Reporting on the work of the illustration firm Anatomical Travelogue Inc. in 2003, TIME writer Jyoti Thottam compared the firm's artists and programmers to "monks in a scriptorium, lined up at superfast HP workstations . . . Their manuscripts are digital scans of the body, illuminated into images so startlingly vivid that even scientists stop and stare. And the abbot here is an artist, self-taught in math, physics and business, named Alexander Tsiaras."

Five years later, Tsiaras' firm continues to produce cutting-edge images of the human body that bring our understanding of this infinitely complex organism into sharp and revealing focus. The work involves collecting data from MRI scans, spiral CT scans and other medical imaging technologies and using them to create scientifically faithful 3-D pictures and animations.

The firm's work resists easy categorization, but Tsiaras takes a good stab at it: "It's Pixar meets the National Institutes of Health." Small wonder that when TIME Books began considering the publication of a volume exploring the wonders of the human body, the group's exceptional work seemed the perfect way to illustrate it.

This volume represents a collaboration between TIME's dedicated team of science writers and reporters and the visualization artists of Anatomical Travelogue. It also contains a number of illustrations by TIME's own staff of award-winning graphic designers. Readers who enjoy the Anatomical Travelogue illustrations will also enjoy two books showcasing them: *From Conception to Birth: A Life Unfolds* (Doubleday; 2002) and *The Architecture and Design of Man and Woman* (Doubleday; 2004).

In the fall of 2008, Tsiaras and his team will go online with their most ambitious project yet: TheVisualMD.com is a website designed to present the most up-to-date and scientifically accurate 3-D depictions of the human body ever made available to both lay people and professionals. Tsiaras intends the new site to be a "richly visual interactive experience on the Web that will demystify disease for participants, enable them to understand its causes and consequences and offer them pathways back to health." It's an ambitious dream, but one expects an abbot of digits to pursue lofty visions.

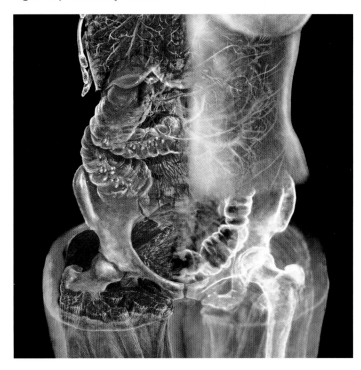

Insights *Anatomical Travelogue artists use state-of-the-art imaging tools, such as magnetic resonance imaging (MRI) and computerized tomography (CT), to compile digital slices of the body. These individual slices are then translated into the three-dimensional models. The digital sections are processed through several steps, including the isolation of segments that make up cells, tissues, organs, systems and pathologies; the examination in 3-D of details of anatomical structures; and the visual highlighting of areas of interest through the use of color, opacity and camera angle. The image above shows the range of different segmentations and rendering methods that can be applied to data captured by a CT scan*

contents

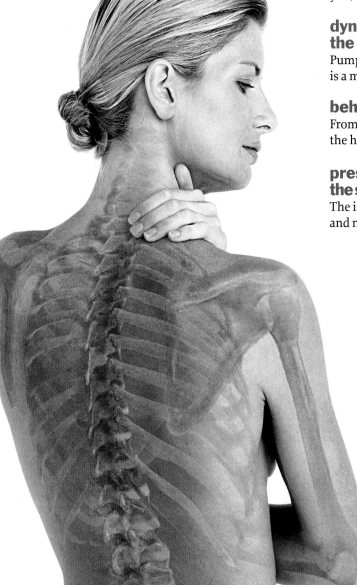

Illuminating the body
From the spine to the lungs to the DNA within each cell, the human body is a marvel of complexity whose internal systems operate through electrical, chemical and physical networks that we are only beginning to understand

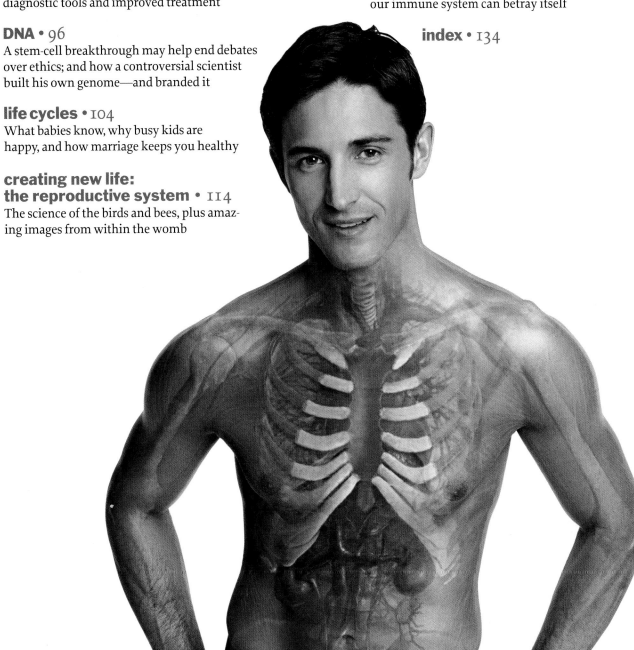

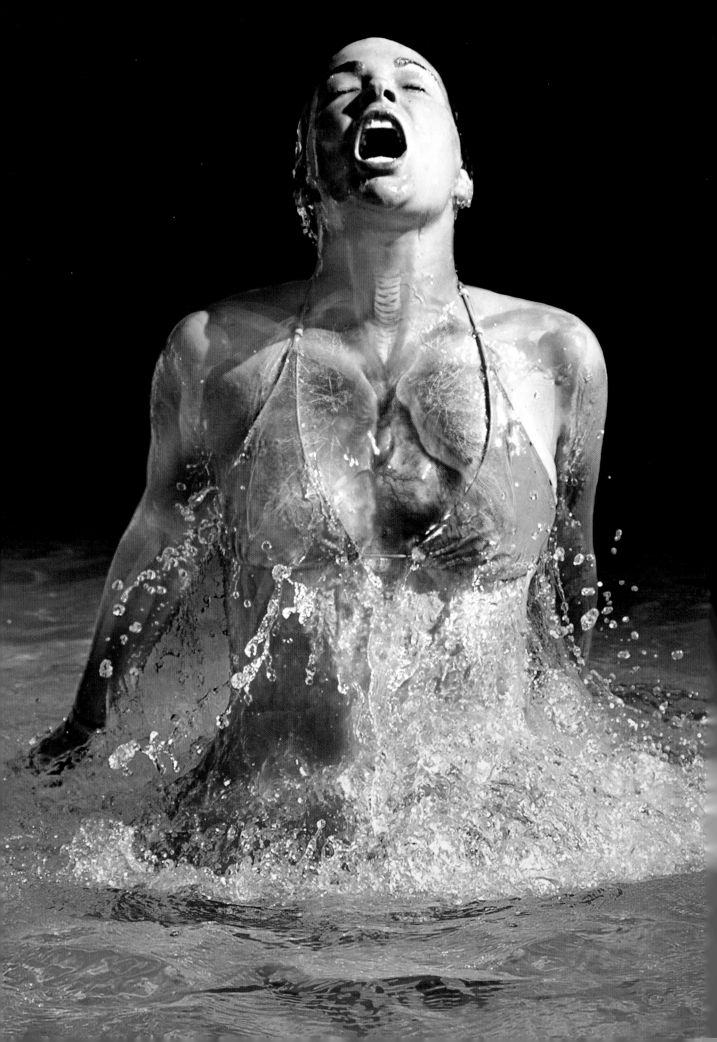

Exploring the Body

HUMAN BEINGS ARE CAPABLE OF AMAZING FEATS: WE CAN GOVERN ourselves, build astounding structures in which to live and work, but above all, we can explore. And our journeys have taken us not only to the outer reaches of space but also to the inner depths of ourselves. As human beings, nothing captivates us more than the human body. The following pages are only the latest record of our quest to explore the body, a chronicle of how genes, cells, tissues, muscle, bone, brain and blood come together to operate as one coherent whole. But this is a journey whose story does not have a neat beginning, middle and end: it is a learning experience that is constantly evolving. Even things we thought we knew, such as the number of genes strung together in the human genome, needed adjusting once we figured out a way to sequence our DNA (it turns out we have about 30,000 genes, not 140,000, as scientists had originally believed). Sophisticated imaging techniques have helped us appreciate that heart attacks are not simply the result of fatty plaques clogging up blood vessels; they are a by-product of the deadly union between inflammation and those plaques. Our understanding of what goes wrong when diseases such as cancer and dementia strike is also in flux, offering flashes of insight that help us stock our pharmacy shelves with better and safer medicines and develop faster, more accurate ways of knowing when the exquisite machinery of the human body starts to falter. So revel in the journey that unfolds in the following chapters, keeping in mind that as much as we know about the human body, the odyssey is just beginning. ■

—Alice Park

Breath of life *Our first act upon emerging into the world is to take a huge, gulping breath, and once we do, we can't stop. It's our way of stripping the oxygen out of the air and depositing this life-sustaining gas into our blood, and the lungs are the bellows that make it all happen. So take a deep breath— and keep your body's essential air-pump working*

Fluid motion *Even underwater, the 200 bones of the skeleton provide both shape and support for the body. They also serve as anchors for the powerful muscles that contract and release to propel a swimmer through the water. And as strong as they are, bones are also surprisingly light, giving our muscles the ability to keep us buoyant and bobbing around when we find ourselves submerged. Even less obvious are bones' hidden talents: red marrow, a rich fluid that courses through bones of the arms and legs, constantly churns out the red blood cells that carry oxygen throughout the body, while other parts of bone produce the white blood cells that defend us against foreign invaders such as viruses and bacteria.*

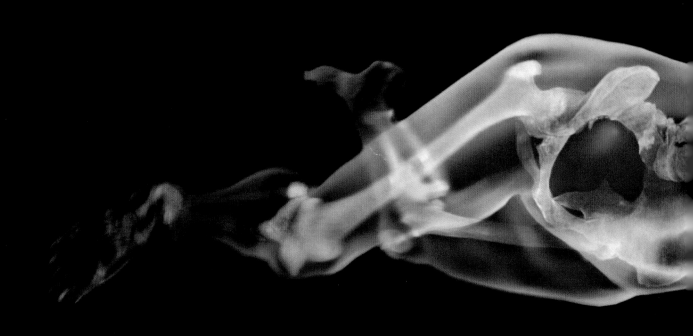

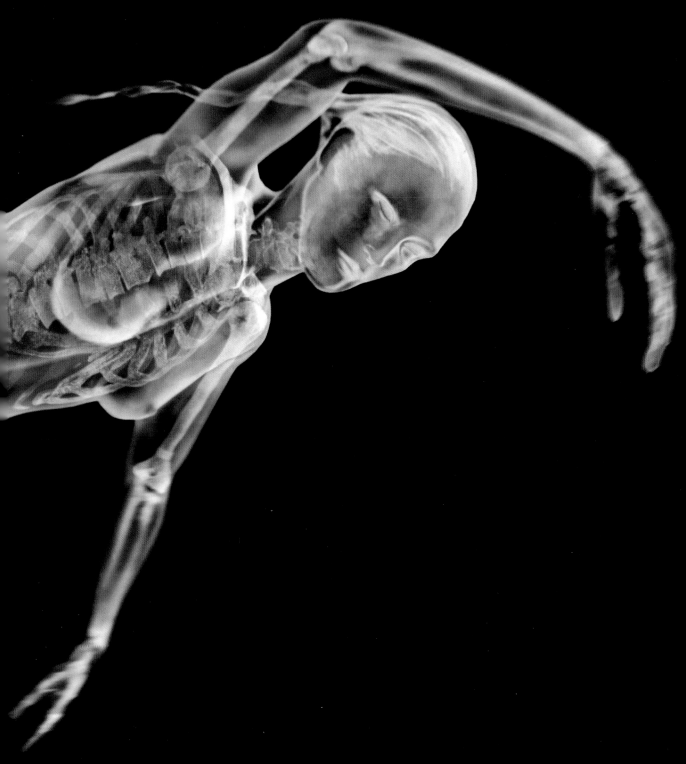

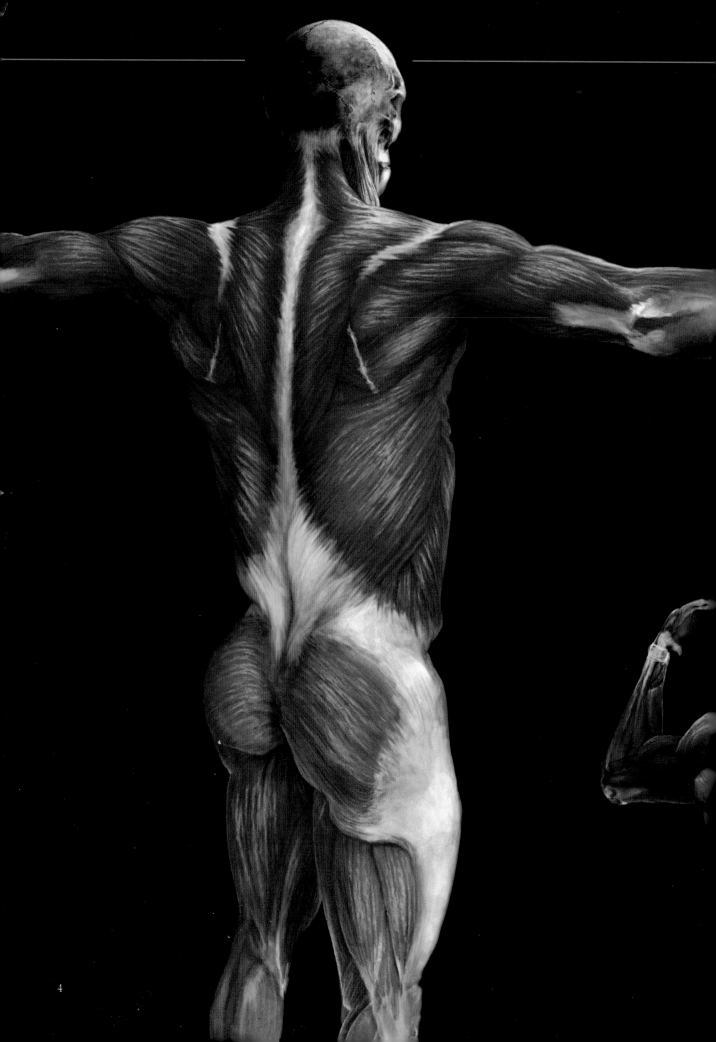

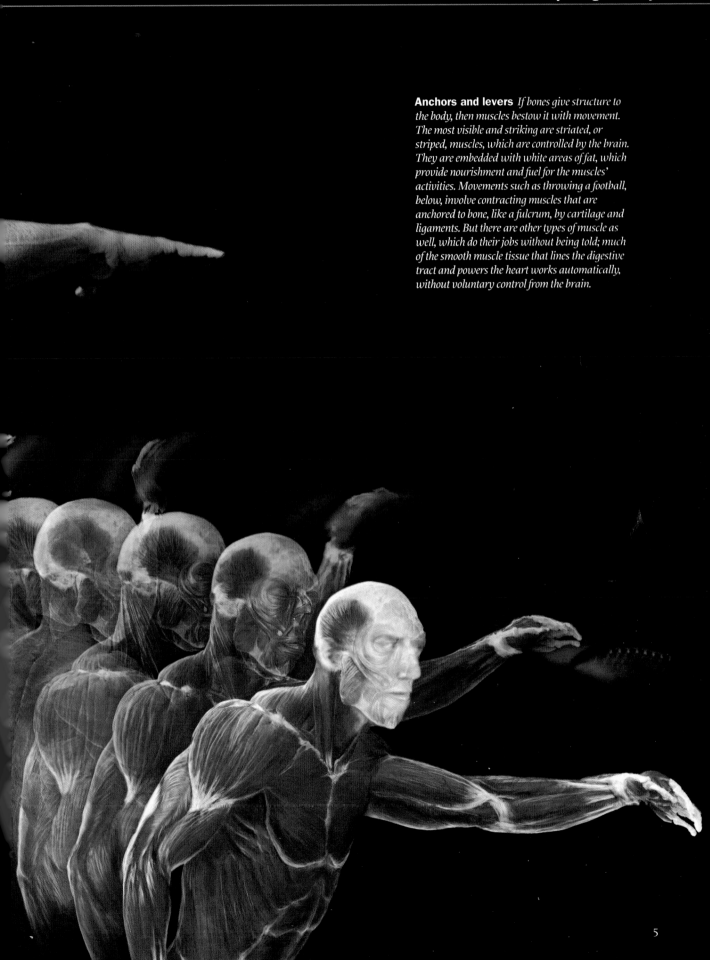

Anchors and levers *If bones give structure to the body, then muscles bestow it with movement. The most visible and striking are striated, or striped, muscles, which are controlled by the brain. They are embedded with white areas of fat, which provide nourishment and fuel for the muscles' activities. Movements such as throwing a football, below, involve contracting muscles that are anchored to bone, like a fulcrum, by cartilage and ligaments. But there are other types of muscle as well, which do their jobs without being told; much of the smooth muscle tissue that lines the digestive tract and powers the heart works automatically, without voluntary control from the brain.*

5

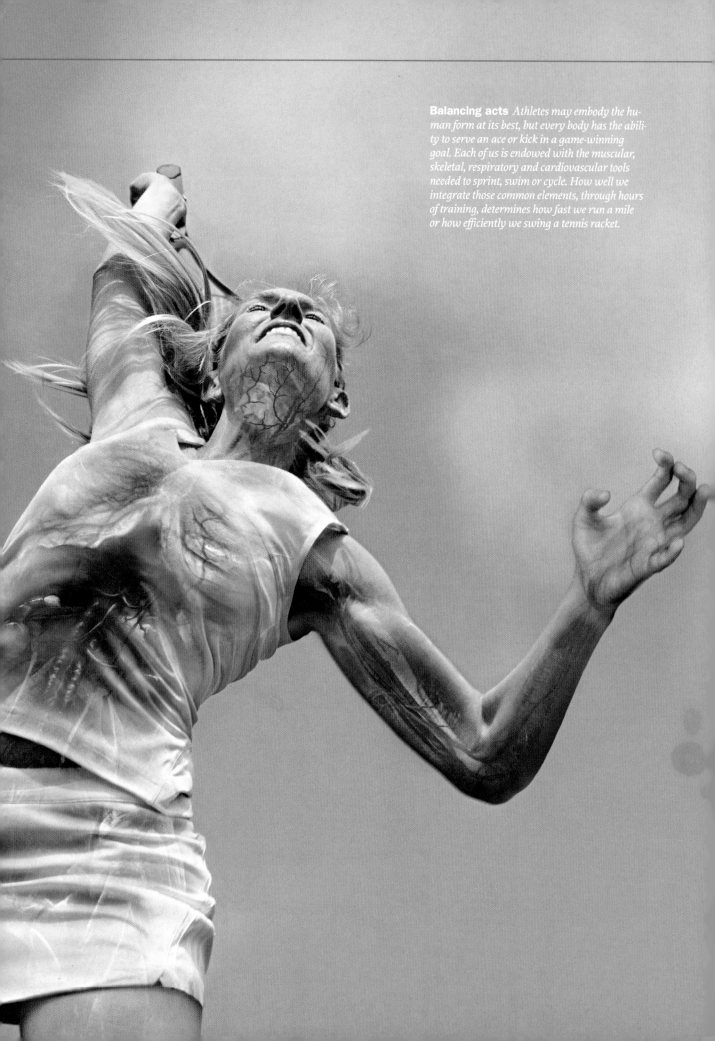

Balancing acts *Athletes may embody the human form at its best, but every body has the ability to serve an ace or kick in a game-winning goal. Each of us is endowed with the muscular, skeletal, respiratory and cardiovascular tools needed to sprint, swim or cycle. How well we integrate those common elements, through hours of training, determines how fast we run a mile or how efficiently we swing a tennis racket.*

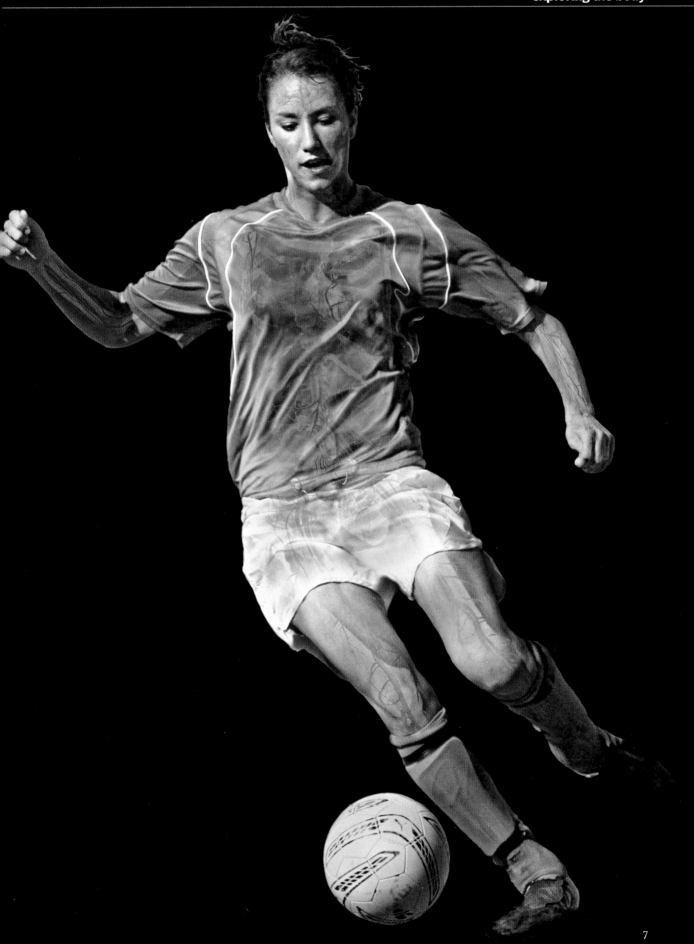

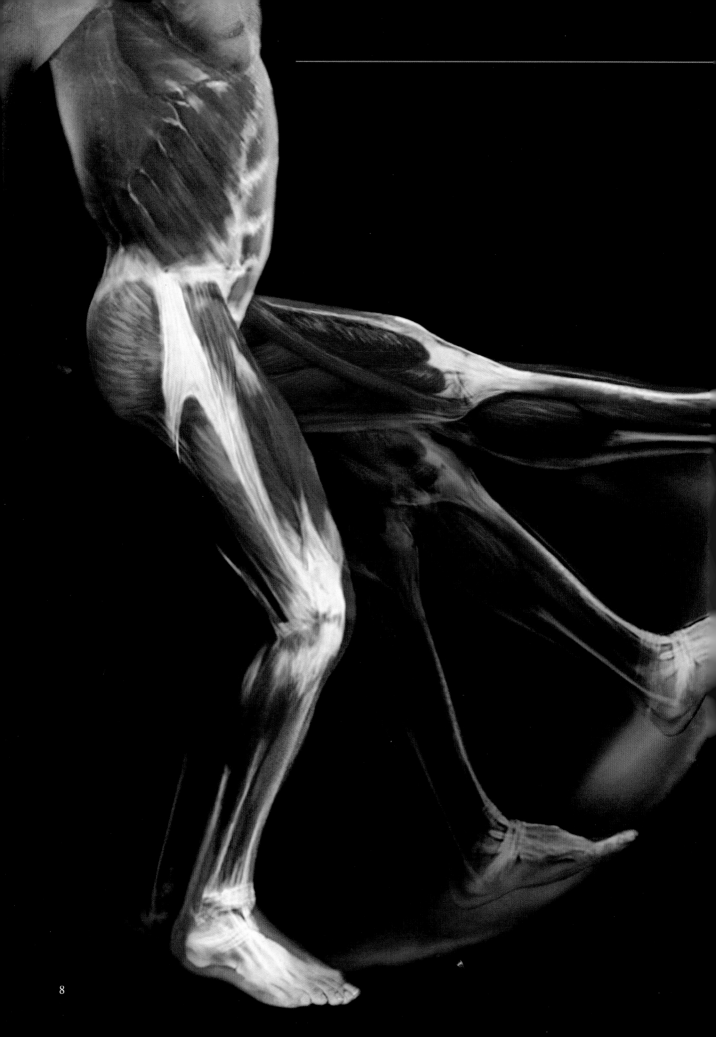

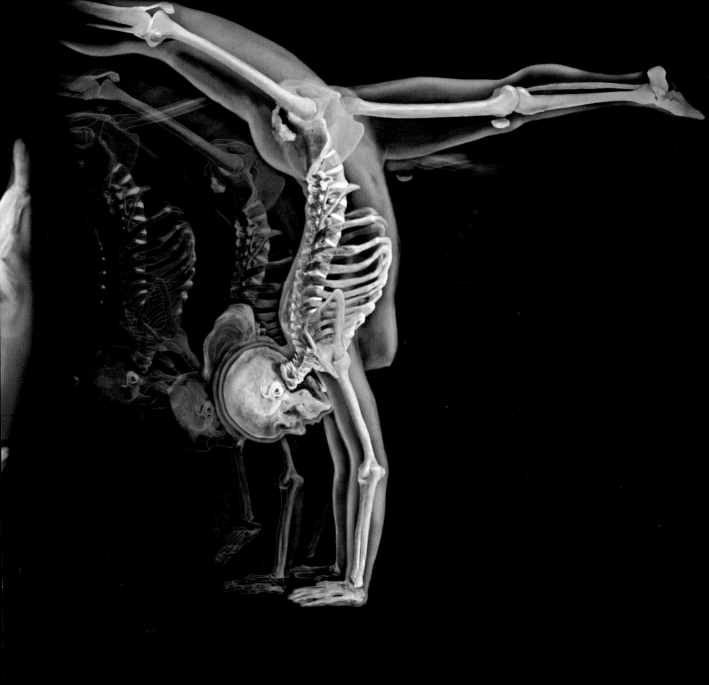

Human endurance *Big or small, every movement requires an exquisite choreography of push and pull, contraction and release. Kicking a ball centers around the femur, or thighbone, the longest bone in the body, and the knee. Because of the femur's length, the blood vessels feeding it and the hamstring and quadriceps muscles responsible for moving it are also among the body's longest. With all of this power centralized on the relatively smaller knee, it's no wonder that the ligaments holding this critical joint together can tear so easily.*

Coordinating all of this muscular ballet to ensure that every movement is balanced out in a smooth final motion are a series of tiny structures nestled deep in the inner ear. Two sets of fluid-filled organs, the utricle and saccule, register the position of the head, while three semicircular canals, set at right angles to one another, pick up rotational movement to keep us balanced, even if we're upside down and on our hands.

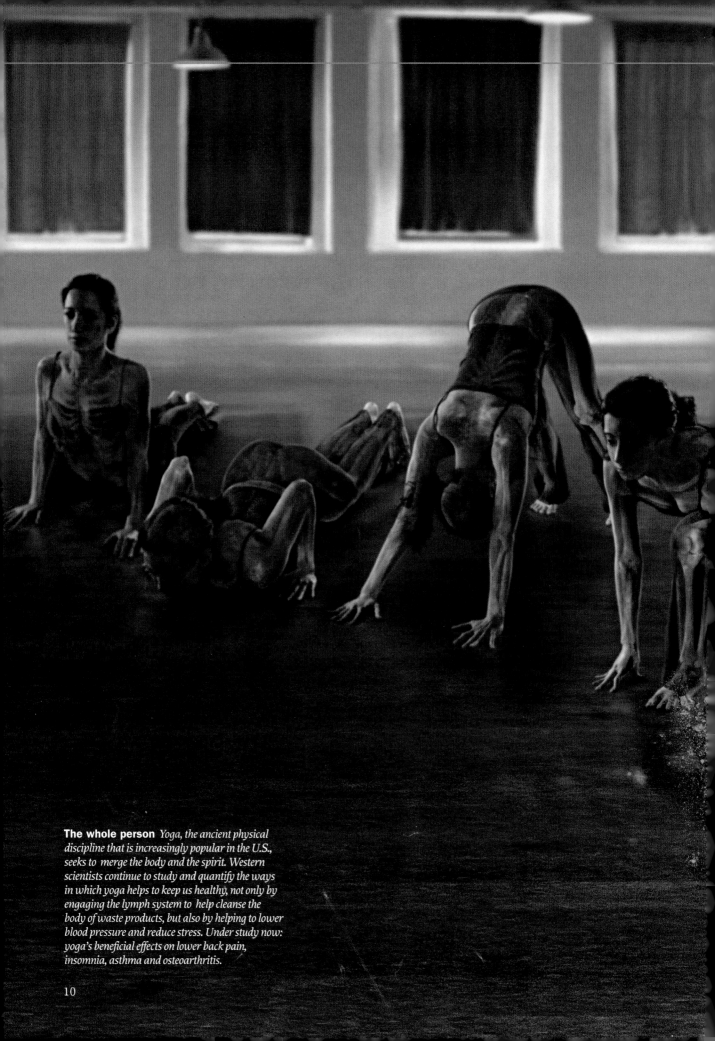

The whole person *Yoga, the ancient physical discipline that is increasingly popular in the U.S., seeks to merge the body and the spirit. Western scientists continue to study and quantify the ways in which yoga helps to keep us healthy, not only by engaging the lymph system to help cleanse the body of waste products, but also by helping to lower blood pressure and reduce stress. Under study now: yoga's beneficial effects on lower back pain, insomnia, asthma and osteoarthritis.*

10

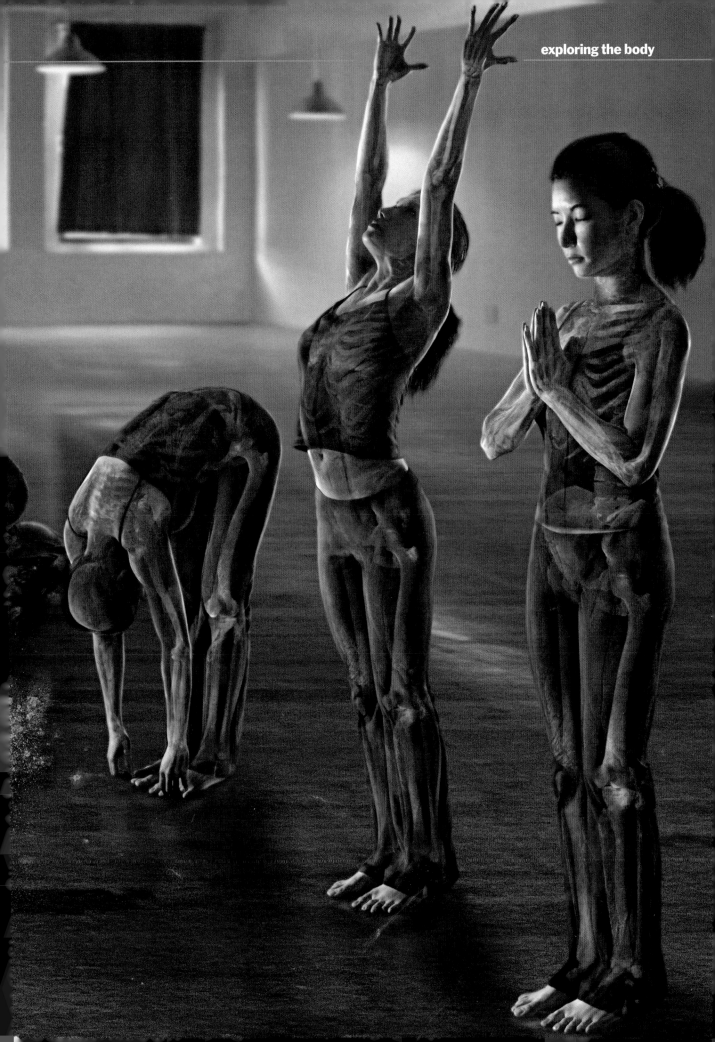

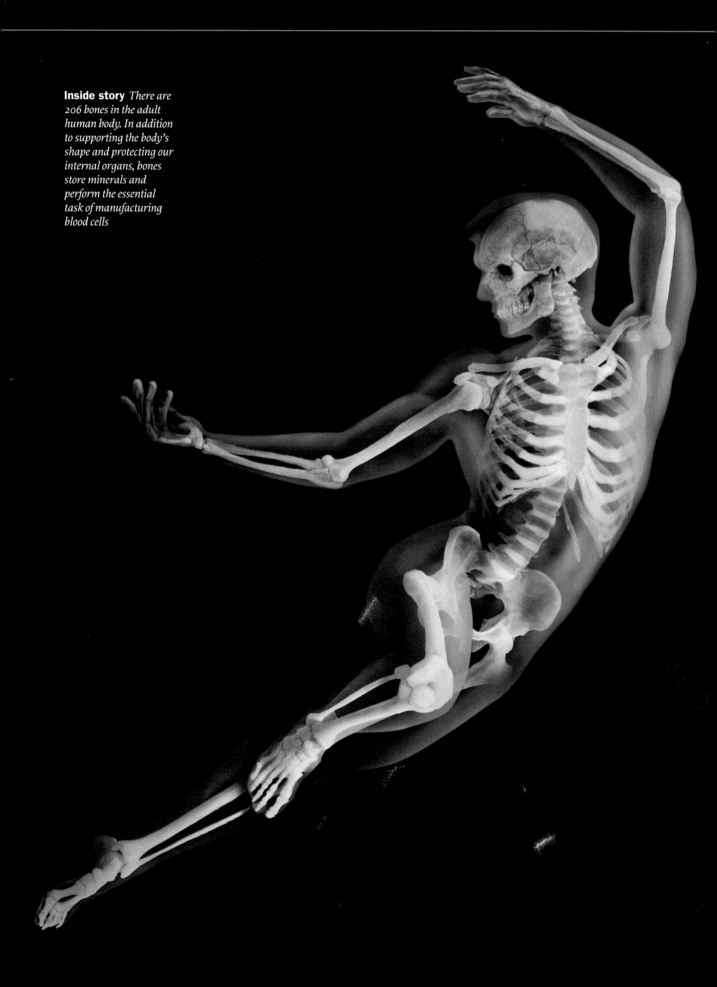

Inside story *There are 206 bones in the adult human body. In addition to supporting the body's shape and protecting our internal organs, bones store minerals and perform the essential task of manufacturing blood cells*

Bone and Brawn

Shape, support, movement: the skeletal and muscular systems

I T'S IRONIC THAT OUR FOLKLORE HAS COME TO ASSOCI-ate skeletons with mortality. Bones are indeed the pieces of us that endure longest in a grave, continuing to stave off decay months and years after softer tissues have disappeared. Yet it is bones that also speak to us about human history across countless millenniums, providing scientists with evidence and insights that bring the world of our ancestors to life.

Rather than embodying human frailty, our skeletons are the strongest things about us. Many bones are able to withstand thousands of pounds of force per square inch. Indeed, Henry Gray's classic 1918 text, *Anatomy of the Human Body*, contains a chart showing that bone is, in most cases, tougher than both oak and granite, although slightly less strong than steel. And that's all the more remarkable considering that bone is a living tissue.

Even when we reach adulthood, our skeletal system is not physiologically complete. Instead, our bones are constantly being built up and torn down, like a house under constant renovation. That's why broken or fractured bones can heal so seamlessly, and also why exercises like walking or jogging are good for us: they stimulate the production of fresh bone tissue. But if bones are inactive too long, all that building up starts to slow down, reducing bone mass, which leads to a corresponding loss of strength and mobility. It's the same effect seen in astronauts, who suffer bone loss after prolonged periods of low gravity in Earth orbit, although the condition can be quickly reversed by vigorous activity once the astronauts are safely back on Planet Earth.

If bones are the hardware of the body's mobility, muscles, joints and cartilage are the software that connects and moves our body parts. All but one of the bones in the human skeleton connect to others at more than 100 joints, which fall into half a dozen separate types of design: bones hinge, pivot and glide where they meet. Propelled by surrounding muscle, our bones and joints are capable of 16 different types of motion, including rotation, extension and abduction. Simply wiggling your fingers can involve as many as six of these motions at once, employing dozens of separate bones and muscles.

Some anthropologists believe that the emergence of the saddle joint at the base of each thumb defines us as human beings more than any of the more complex systems in our bodies. This opposable thumb, capable of moving against the palm and other fingers, was, in this view, the evolutionary spark that led to developments like tools, technology and the larger brain needed to manage them. ■

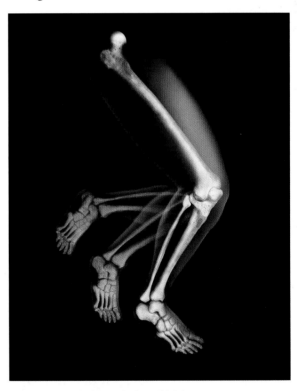

Hinge joint *The femur, the long thigh bone, connects to the lower leg at one of the most complex junctions in the body, the knee joint*

Anatomy Lesson Bones

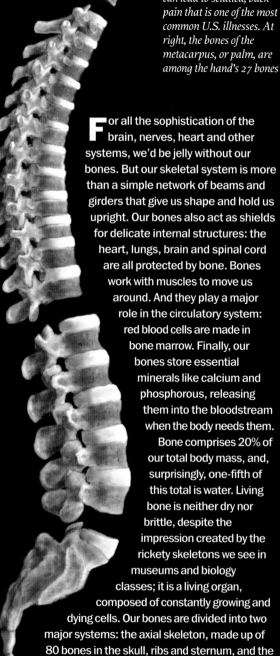

Pillars of stability *The spine, left, consists of 33 vertebrae that protect the spinal cord within them. Problems with the disks that cushion the vertebrae can lead to sciatica, back pain that is one of the most common U.S. illnesses. At right, the bones of the metacarpus, or palm, are among the hand's 27 bones*

For all the sophistication of the brain, nerves, heart and other systems, we'd be jelly without our bones. But our skeletal system is more than a simple network of beams and girders that give us shape and hold us upright. Our bones also act as shields for delicate internal structures: the heart, lungs, brain and spinal cord are all protected by bone. Bones work with muscles to move us around. And they play a major role in the circulatory system: red blood cells are made in bone marrow. Finally, our bones store essential minerals like calcium and phosphorous, releasing them into the bloodstream when the body needs them. Bone comprises 20% of our total body mass, and, surprisingly, one-fifth of this total is water. Living bone is neither dry nor brittle, despite the impression created by the rickety skeletons we see in museums and biology classes; it is a living organ, composed of constantly growing and dying cells. Our bones are divided into two major systems: the axial skeleton, made up of 80 bones in the skull, ribs and sternum, and the appendicular skeleton, which contains 126 bones in the shoulders, limbs and pelvis. In a woman, the pelvis is wider and shallower than a man's, to allow for childbirth. Bones fall into four categories, depending on their shape: long bones such as the femur, or thigh bone; short bones, including the metacarpals in the hand; flat bones, such as the sternum, or chest bone; and, finally, the irregular bones, which includes the vertebrae.

Although many people imagine that bones are mostly static, they are actually a beehive of microscopic activity, with three types of cells constantly at work. Osteocytes maintain healthy bone tissue, taking in nutrients from the bloodstream and recycling waste materials. Osteoblasts build new bone tissue while we are young and repair damaged bones in maturity. Osteoclasts regulate bone growth.

More than half of the 200-plus bones in our bodies are devoted to a pair of distinctly human activities: we walk upright thanks to our feet, which contain (between them) 52 bones, while our ability to manipulate our environment is made possible by the 54 separate bones in our hands.

Less sturdy but equally critical bones help us to hear and speak: the ossicle bones of the middle ear, known informally as the "hammer," "anvil" and "stirrup," help make human hearing sensitive enough to distinguish among some 40,000 distinct sounds. And human speech is made possible by the hyoid bone in the neck, which floats freely in soft tissue and enables the movements and vibrations of the tongue, pharynx and larynx to produce the wide variety of sounds we know as talking. To perform this remarkable function, the hyoid is the only piece of the human skeleton that is not attached to any other bone.

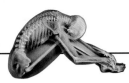

Common Muscoloskeletal Diseases and Disorders

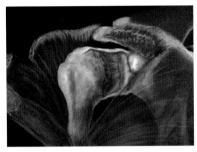 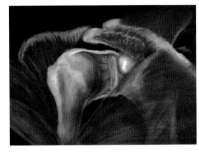

Arthritis and joints *Arthritis attacks the joints and can take various forms. At left is a healthy shoulder joint; at right is a joint whose cartilage is breaking down due to calcium deposits whose buildup leaves the bone exposed and looking "punched out" and eroded*

Bone Cancer Includes three conditions: osteosarcoma develops in growing bones, usually before age 25; chondrosarcoma begins in cartilage, often after age 50; Ewing's sarcoma develops in nerve tissue in the bone marrow of young people.

■ **Symptoms** *Persistent or unusual pain or swelling in or near a bone is the most common symptom, but not all bone cancers cause pain.*

■ **Treatment** Surgery, chemotherapy, radiation, amputation.

Muscular Dystrophy A group of more than 30 inherited diseases that cause muscle weakness and loss of tissue.

■ **Symptoms** *Vary widely but often include stumbling, waddling, difficulty climbing stairs or standing after sitting.*

■ **Treatment** Physical and speech therapy, orthopedic devices, surgery and medications.

Osteoarthritis Also known as degenerative joint disease, this most common form of arthritis is caused by the breakdown of cartilage in the joints.

■ **Symptoms** *Pain, swelling and reduced motion in the joints, most often in the hands, knees, hips or spine.*

■ **Treatment** There is no cure; therapies include exercise, weight control, rest, pain relief and surgery.

Osteoporosis Also known as porous bone; low bone mass and structural deterioration of bone tissue lead to weakened bone and higher risk of fractures of the hip, spine and wrist.

■ **Symptoms** *Sometimes called the "silent disease," since bone loss occurs without symptoms. Early signs include sagging posture, collapsed vertebrae and, in advanced cases, hip fracture.*

■ **Treatment** Change in diet to increase calcium intake, exercise to reduce weight and increase bone strength and lifestyle modification to prevent fall. Medications can keep bone growing at a healthy rate.

Tendinitis Inflammation of the cords of tissue that attach muscles to bones—commonly caused by exertion but sometimes indicating a more serious underlying condition, such as rheumatoid arthritis.

■ **Symptoms** *Pain and tenderness near a joint; most often in the shoulders, elbows, knees, hips, heels or wrists.*

■ **Treatment** Rest; application of ice and medications to relieve pain and decrease swelling; physical therapy; steroid injections; surgery.

Source: National Institutes of Health

Weak bones *Osteoporosis can lead to weakening of the spine, resulting in deteriorating posture*

The Bones
Terms to Know

Axial skeleton The 80 bones of the skull, ribs and sternum that form the vertical axis of the body.

Appendicular skeleton The 126 bones of the shoulders, limbs and pelvis that form our appendages and their attachments to the axial skeleton.

Bone density/Bone mass Measures of the amount of calcium contained in a given volume of bone.

Calcium Mineral that helps form bones and maintain their strength. Most calcium is stored in your bones and teeth.

Collagen A family of stiff, helical, insoluble protein macromolecules that function as scaffolding and provide tensile strength in fibrous tissues and rigidity in bone.

Osteoblasts Cells that form new bone matter.

Osteoclasts Bone-resorbing cells.

Osteocytes The cells of established bone.

Periosteum A sleeve of connective tissue that surrounds the shaft of the bone and contributes to fracture healing.

Vitamin D The nutrient that helps the body absorb calcium, most often supplied by milk, tuna fish or eggs and moderate exposure to sunlight.

Sources: American Academy of Orthopaedic Surgeons; Centers for Disease Control; National Institutes of Health

■ On the Horizon Briefs

One Bad Back, Two Cures Both surgery and therapy can help those with severe back pain

Back pain is one of the leading causes of workplace absenteeism and is the fifth leading cause of expenditures in U.S. hospitals each year. One of the most common sources of back woes is sciatica, caused by a herniated, slipped or protruding disc that impinges on the sciatic nerve, sending pain down the leg.

The pain of sciatica can be unbearable, leading patients to take multiple pain medications—and to seek a quick surgical fix. Around the world, some 1.5 million people each year undergo operations to relieve pressure on the sciatic nerve, a procedure that usually brings them the relief they seek. But new research suggests that over the course of time, surgery may be no better than nonoperative therapeutic methods.

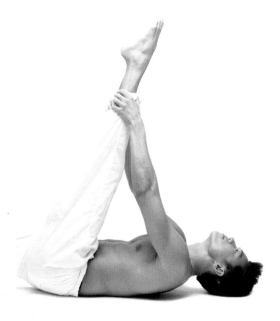

In a 2007 study published in the *New England Journal of Medicine,* researchers followed 283 patients who had suffered with sciatic pain for at least six weeks. Half of them were scheduled for surgery, and the other half underwent conservative treatments—principally rest, gentle stretching and back-strengthening exercises and, when needed, anti-inflammatories. Some 95% of participants in both groups reported significant recovery after one year. That's good news for those concerned about surgical risks, which can include bleeding or even accidental nerve damage that may only exacerbate the pain. What's more, surgery can cost a few thousand dollars and requires months for full recovery.

Osteo Woes A new osteoporosis drug arrives—with a warning

For most folks, drinking plenty of milk and getting enough vitamin D and exercise are sufficient to keep bones strong. But for some people, additional bone-building is needed. Zoledronic acid, marketed as Reclast, is the first once-a-year treatment approved for osteoporosis in postmenopausal women. It can also be prescribed for both sexes to treat the bone disorder Paget's disease.

But you might not want to jump too fast for the annual IV infusion. Like most drugs, Reclast comes with side effects, and the FDA is reviewing data showing that it and other osteoporosis medications may increase abnormal heart rhythms.

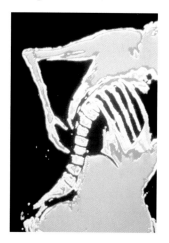

Prosthetics A timely advance in creating artificial limbs

Nothing replaces the body parts you were born with, but technology is making artificial limbs steadily better—and just in time. In part because of the growing number of wounded vets returning from Iraq, the population of amputees living in the U.S. will increase 42% by 2020. Scientists at Johns Hopkins University have developed a revolutionary prototype for a prosthetic hand, below, that lets the user grip objects by connecting remaining nerves near the injury with unused muscles that can then flex and operate the hand.

Meanwhile, Hanger Orthopedic Group in Bethesda, Md., has developed a suction-producing gel that helps prosthetics wearers comfortably hold the fake limb in place, enhancing the traditional stump-and-socket attachment, which can cause painful skin infections.

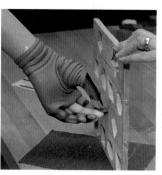

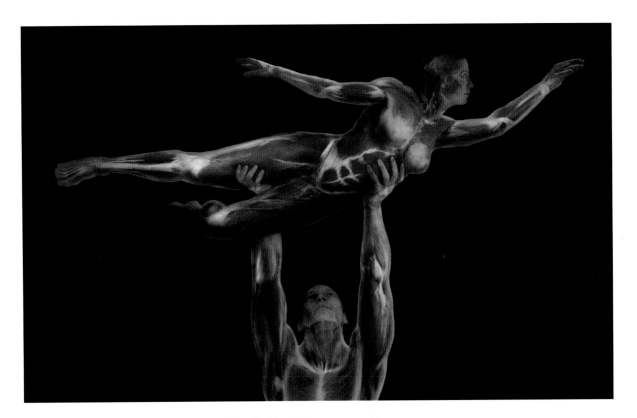

Contractual Obligations The muscle system

READ THIS BOOK FOR 60 MINUTES, AND THE MUSCLES around your eye will contract more than 10,000 times. If something you see in these pages causes you to smile, you will need 17 facial muscles to do so. If anything provokes a frown, that will activate 42 muscles in the face and neck. Get up and walk across the room, and more than 200 muscles will fire. Feeling tired yet?

The human body contains between 600 and 800 muscles, depending on which system of counting you choose, and they account for between a quarter and half of your total body mass, depending on your size and body type. Either way, we all carry around three kinds of muscle: skeletal, smooth and cardiac. Skeletal muscles primarily join bones together and are mostly controlled by conscious thought. Smooth muscles are found inside internal organs and in the walls of veins and arteries; they are controlled by involuntary brain processes. Cardiac muscle is found only in the heart.

Your muscles are always at work. The muscles of the heart, eyes and mouth are the body's busiest. While the heart twitches more than 100,000 times each day, the muscle groups around (and inside) your eyes nearly equal this total—and might exceed it if our eyes did not become mostly inactive during the hours we sleep. And the tongue, operated by a group of 16 muscles, works around the clock: active not only when we eat and speak, it also aids in breathing and is constantly pushing saliva down our throats, even when we sleep.

All muscles work by contracting. Despite what our body tells us is happening, not one of them can push on anything. Rather, they achieve this task by contracting around the outside of joints that act as fulcrums. When push comes to shove, the biceps on the inside of your upper arm contract, as if to pull a stuck door toward you, and your triceps on the outside contracts from the opposite direction, swinging your forearm outward and allowing you to apply force against the door.

Muscles do more than move us and hold us together; they also play a vital role in maintaining our internal body temperature. In truth, only about one-fourth of all the energy generated by muscles goes to movement. The rest is radiated as heat, which the body recycles back through all its tissues. When our body temperature drops too low, the brain kicks several muscle groups into overdrive, attempting to generate heat by the rapid vibrating movement we know as shivering. ■

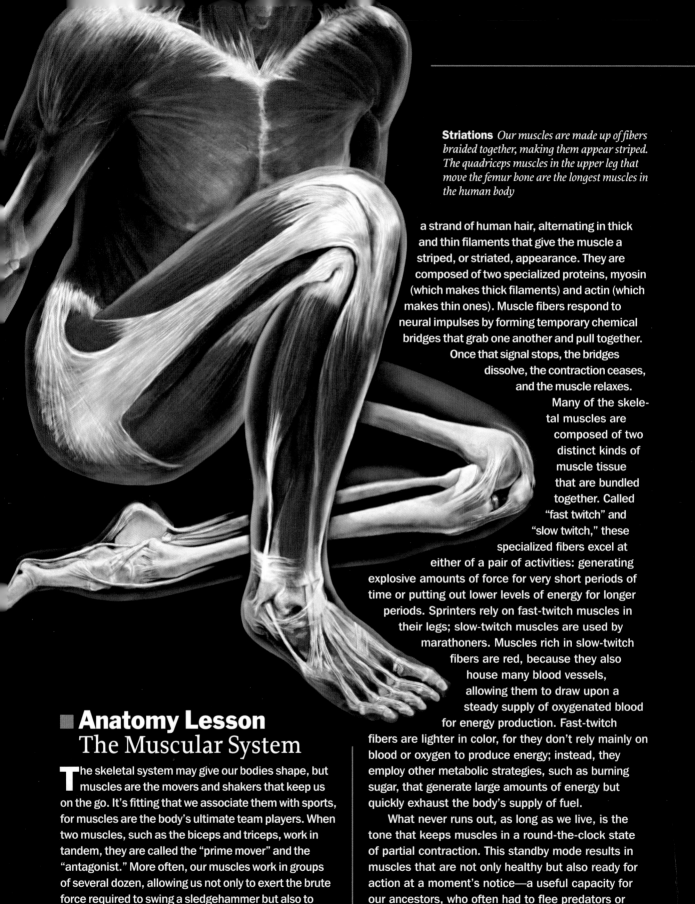

a strand of human hair, alternating in thick and thin filaments that give the muscle a striped, or striated, appearance. They are composed of two specialized proteins, myosin (which makes thick filaments) and actin (which makes thin ones). Muscle fibers respond to neural impulses by forming temporary chemical bridges that grab one another and pull together. Once that signal stops, the bridges dissolve, the contraction ceases, and the muscle relaxes.

Many of the skeletal muscles are composed of two distinct kinds of muscle tissue that are bundled together. Called "fast twitch" and "slow twitch," these specialized fibers excel at either of a pair of activities: generating explosive amounts of force for very short periods of time or putting out lower levels of energy for longer periods. Sprinters rely on fast-twitch muscles in their legs; slow-twitch muscles are used by marathoners. Muscles rich in slow-twitch fibers are red, because they also house many blood vessels, allowing them to draw upon a steady supply of oxygenated blood for energy production. Fast-twitch fibers are lighter in color, for they don't rely mainly on blood or oxygen to produce energy; instead, they employ other metabolic strategies, such as burning sugar, that generate large amounts of energy but quickly exhaust the body's supply of fuel.

What never runs out, as long as we live, is the tone that keeps muscles in a round-the-clock state of partial contraction. This standby mode results in muscles that are not only healthy but also ready for action at a moment's notice—a useful capacity for our ancestors, who often had to flee predators or chase prey with little warning. Muscle tone and the operation of the cardiac muscles in our heart are the only functions of our muscular system that are beyond our voluntary control.

■ Anatomy Lesson
The Muscular System

The skeletal system may give our bodies shape, but muscles are the movers and shakers that keep us on the go. It's fitting that we associate them with sports, for muscles are the body's ultimate team players. When two muscles, such as the biceps and triceps, work in tandem, they are called the "prime mover" and the "antagonist." More often, our muscles work in groups of several dozen, allowing us not only to exert the brute force required to swing a sledgehammer but also to achieve the precise gradations of tension needed to tease a Chopin nocturne out of a piano.

Tissue in the skeletal muscles, those we consciously control, is composed of fibers many times thinner than

Muscles Terms to Know

Anabolic steroids Synthetic analogs of testosterone; can be used to enhance muscle-building effects in athletes.

Anaerobic metabolism Oxygen debt; when the cardiovascular system is unable to meet the needs of working muscles, anaerobic metabolism is activated.

Extensor A muscle that acts to make a limb assume a more straight line; the antagonist of a flexor.

Flexor A muscle that acts to flex or bend a joint.

Inflammation Heat, redness, swelling and pain that accompany musculoskeletal injuries when tissue is crushed, stretched or torn.

Ligament A collagenous tissue that connects two bones at a joint.

Quadriceps contusion Muscle soreness and stiffness caused by overstrain or a contusion; also known as a "charley horse."

Range of motion The amount of movement available at a joint.

Sarcopenia Loss of muscle mass and strength as a result of aging.

Tendon Tough, ropelike fibrous tissue that attaches muscle to bone and transmits forces of contraction.

Source: American Academy of Orthopaedic Surgeons

A Plague of ACL Injuries for Female Athletes

In recent years, female athletes have experienced a huge uptick in serious knee injuries, especially tearing of the anterior cruciate ligament (ACL). That's the type of damage in which the ligament detaches from the femur bone. In adults, correcting the problem usually requires surgery to reconstruct the ligament. According to a study of NCAA athletes, the tears occur at least twice as often—and in some sports up to eight times as often—in female as in male athletes.

Researchers at the Cleveland Clinic recently tried to better understand how these injuries happen and what makes them different in men and women. Using motion-sensor cameras to capture joint movements, the scientists were able to reconstruct the biomechanics of athletes as they performed drop landings from a 40-cm hang bar. What they discovered is that when the athletes first start jumping, the women are more likely to land on their feet in ways that make them vulnerable to ACL tears. The distance between their knees is narrower, the ankle is more flexed, and the foot rolls outward more. But when either men or women are fatigued, they tend to make those same mistakes, putting both groups at high risk for the painful injury.

What we can all learn from the study is that the body needs to be prepared for when it becomes fatigued by an activity. That means paying extra attention to posture, breathing, strength and most important, being aware that you are getting tired while you exercise. Core strengthening also helps improve form, so exercises like sit-ups, crunches, back exercises and planks can be beneficial.

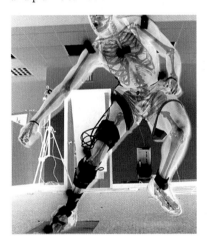

Inner vision

In Search of a Cure for Restless Legs

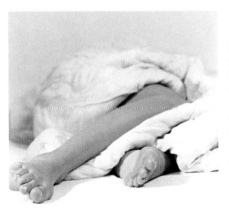

For the estimated 3% of people who experience the prickly, twitchy, downright creepy sensation of the sleep disorder known as restless-leg syndrome (RLS), recent research offers a bit of welcome news. Icelandic scientists studied nearly 1,000 RLS subjects and their family members and traced uncontrolled limb movements, one symptom of the condition, to a gene that regulates the body's iron levels. Studying the gene could help scientists figure out how to shut RLS off at its source.

Scientists have yet to find the precise cause of RLS, but it has been noted that the condition is worsened by stress. The abnormal sensations primarily occur in the lower leg but may also occur in the upper leg, feet or arms. For those afflicted, warm baths, gentle stretching exercises, massage or similar techniques may help alleviate symptoms. At present, there is no cure.

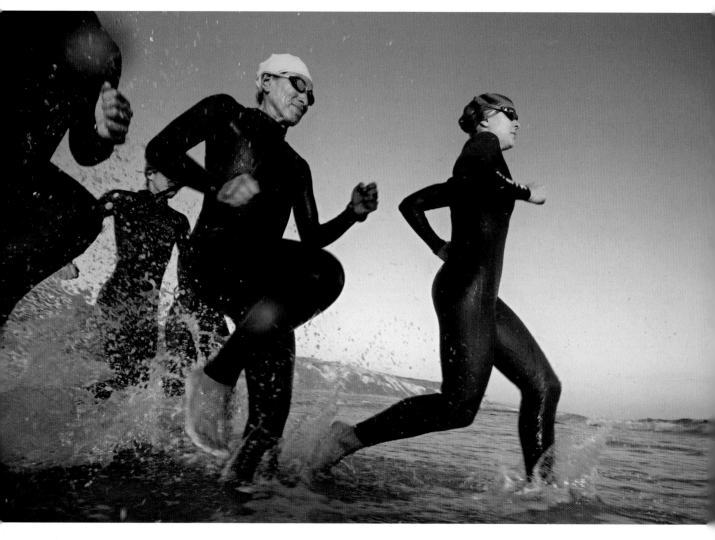

Let's Get a Move On!

Exercise is an essential component of a healthy lifestyle

AMERICANS DIDN'T WORRY MUCH ABOUT KEEPING fit 100 years ago. In those days 40% of the population was reaping and sowing, herding and mowing its way through life on preindustrial farms. In coastal cities, strong-shouldered stevedores were loading and unloading ships dawn to dusk. Builders, lumberjacks and railroad men drove nails or sawed wood using their brawn, not power tools. And for those doing the washing, cooking and scrubbing at home, life wasn't so dainty either. In that bygone, sweat-drenched era, staying active just wasn't an issue. Indoor plumbing? Now that was an issue. Working out? Never heard of it.

One can only imagine what time travelers from that strenuous era would make of modern-day Americans, sitting on their duffs most of the day—in the car, at the office, in school, on the sofa—eating like a stevedore and then driving to the fitness club to log a mile or so on a conveyor belt.

It just doesn't add up. Literally. The old energy-balance equation—calories in should equal calories out—is seriously out of whack, as the rising rates of obesity in the U.S. and other developed nations prove. For much of the past decade, public health officials, doctors and the popular press have focused on the intake side of the equation. We're eating too much fat, too many carbs, too much altogether. But the problem is just as grave on the output

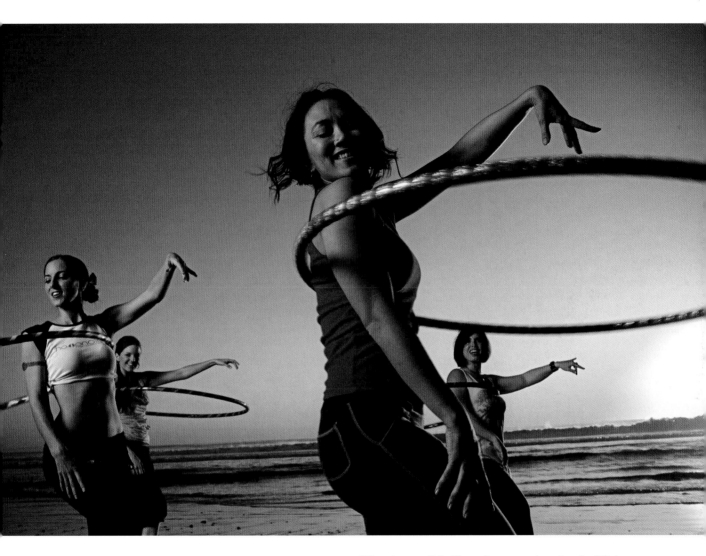

Slim chance *Triathlon swimmers and synchronized Hula Hoopers get plenty of exercise, but most Americans are seriously out of shape*

side. We are simply not burning enough calories or moving our bodies sufficiently to maintain good health.

Why should we be concerned about fitness? Because as bad as it is to be overweight, it may be just as bad to be inactive. In fact, some health authorities believe it's worse. The health risks of obesity—diabetes, heart attack, high blood pressure and certain cancers, among others—are familiar to most Americans, but physical activity confers benefits "above and beyond what it can provide for weight control," says Harold Kohl, lead epidemiologist at the Physical Activity and Health Branch of the Centers for Disease Control and Prevention (CDC).

How does exercise help us? Kohl is happy to count the

ways. To begin with, exercise works wonders for the heart, improving the lipid profile, reducing the risk of heart disease and restoring function after a heart attack. "It helps tremendously in maintaining bone health whether you are young or an older adult," he notes. In addition, it acts to moderate blood pressure in people with hypertension, can significantly relieve depression and anxiety and appears to help maintain cognitive function in old age. Studies show that physical activity may also act to prevent cancers of the breast and prostate, probably by influencing hormone levels, and of the colon, probably by keeping wastes and any carcinogens they contain moving along. Exercise seems to be so beneficial to cancer pa-

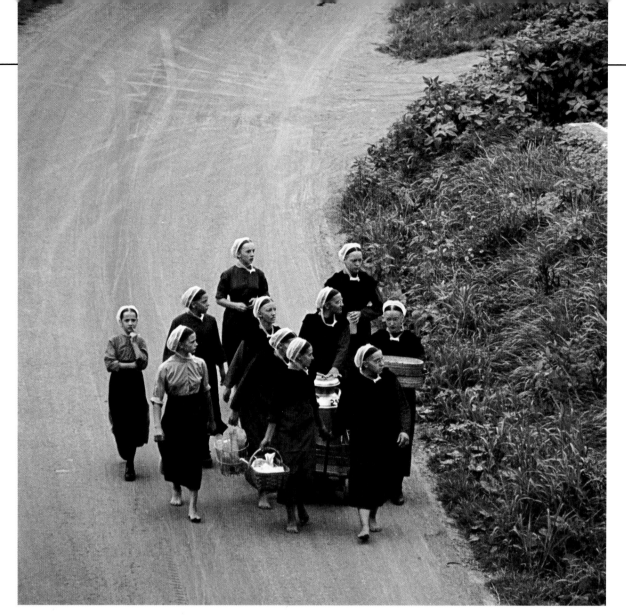

The average Amish man takes 18,245 steps a day, and the average Amish woman takes 14,196. Other Americans, by contrast, take about 5,000

tients that oncologists have begun advising them to do their best to get moving. A 2005 study showed that breast-cancer patients who walked three to five hours a week or did an equivalent amount of another exercise lived about 50% longer than those who were inactive.

Experts cite seven components of fitness, a list that varies a bit from study to study but typically goes something like this: body composition, cardiorespiratory function, flexibility/range of motion, muscle strength, endurance, balance, and agility/coordination. How do Americans stack up on those measures? No one knows. Assessing them requires treadmills, calipers, piles of gym equipment—and lots of money. The President's Council on Physical Fitness and Sports used to conduct a national fitness survey of American schoolkids, but that hasn't happened since the mid-1980s.

What we do know about U.S. fitness comes mainly from measuring body weight and from large polls of individual exercise habits. The signs aren't good. Not only

are nearly a third of American adults obese, but a quarter of them—22% of men, 28% of women—admit that they spend virtually no leisure time getting exercise.

How to get moving? Until mid-2008, most experts recommended getting moderate-to-vigorous exercise 30 min. a day, five days a week. But a new study by University of Pittsburgh researchers found that among a group of women who both dieted and exercised, those who lost 10% of their body weight after two years were exercising just over an hour, five days a week—twice the recommended amount of activity. That doesn't mean health messages about the importance of physical activity were wrong or misguided; the key, doctors say, is to get started with moderate exercise and work your way up to sufficient levels to lose weight and reap your health rewards. As for what moderate means, Kohl offers this guidance: "Walking at about 3 to 3.5 miles per hour is moderate. If you can't maintain a conversation and your heart is beating rapidly, then you've probably crossed into vigorous."

How many of are meeting even the 30-min. standard? In a 2005 TIME survey of more than 1,000 randomly selected American adults, 33% said they do. Federal surveys suggest that it's more like 26%. In short, somewhere from a quarter to half of all Americans say they get the recommended dose of exercise, although the lower figure may be more trustworthy: people are notorious for lying about their exercise habits.

And since the latest evidence seems to be pointing to the need for more, not less exercise, here's a simple, inexpensive way for more of us to get the activity we need: walking. Unfortunately, most American communities were designed in the age of the automobile and aren't built for bipeds. Between 1977 and 1995, trips Americans made by walking declined 40%, even though a quarter of those trips were a mile or less. During the same period, walking to school fell 60%. By 2001 only 13% of trips to school were made by foot or bicycle.

Walking and physical motion have also been steadily drained from the workplace. Americans aren't about to give up their beloved cars and conveniences; if anything, we will continue to eliminate physical effort from our lives. And while a small percentage of the nation—mainly found among the best-educated and wealthiest classes—are committed gym rats, most folks cannot find the time, energy and will power to regularly work out.

To put modern society's lack of movement in context, researchers at the University of Tennessee's Department of Health and Exercise Science studied a group of Old Order Amish, a religious sect that shuns cars and modern machines. Using pedometers, they found that the average Amish man took 18,425 steps a day and the average Amish woman took 14,196 steps. Other gadget-equipped Americans, by contrast, take about 5,000.

Fitness experts increasingly believe that the path to fitness lies in finding new ways to make physical movement an unavoidable part of everyday life. An alliance of public health experts, urban planners and architects is promoting New Urbanism, a movement to build "walkable," mixed-use communities in which residences are close to commercial centers. Such developments are sprouting up, but they remain the exception in 21st-century America. New subdivisions with no place to walk, modern buildings without useable stairways and cash-strapped schools that have dropped P.E. classes remain the rule. The search for a fitter lifestyle for the nation—and for each of us—has to start somewhere, and the best way to do that is to move forward one step at a time. ■

How Americans Exercise

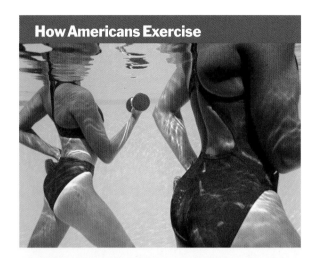

Most Americans say they exercise every week ...

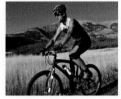

69% take a brisk walk

35% use exercise machines

32% lift weights

30% ride a bike

27% jog or run

22% do aerobics

21% swim

19% dance

18% play a sport

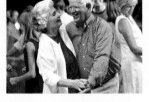

18% go hiking

8% play golf

7% do yoga

7% bowl

And don't forget housework ...

85% work around the house

66% work on the lawn or garden

24% walk or bike on errands

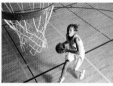

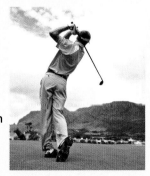

Poll conducted for TIME in 2005 by SRBI Public Affairs

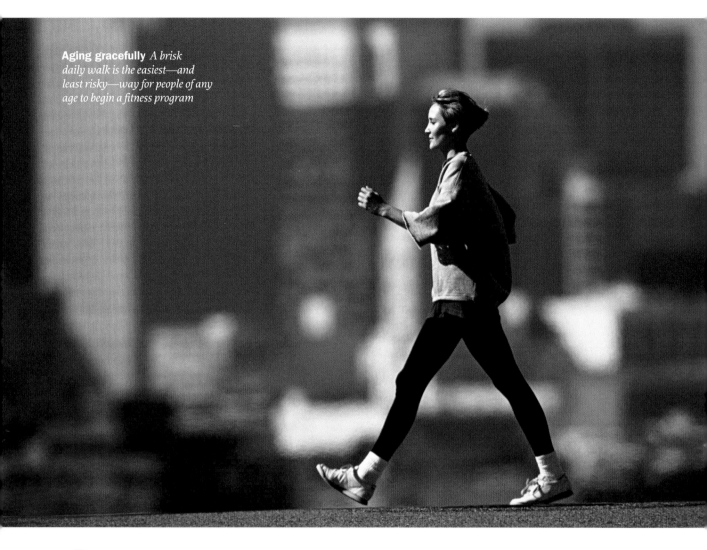

Aging gracefully *A brisk daily walk is the easiest—and least risky—way for people of any age to begin a fitness program*

Couch Potatoes, Arise!

You have nothing to lose but your bulges, so here's how to start

NOTHING IS EASIER THAN FALLING OUT OF SHAPE, especially in the U.S. Americans may no longer lead the world in science, engineering and productivity, but with TiVo on the flat screen, Domino's at the door and an arsenal of remotes within easy reach, we've got leisure time nailed. Climbing off the couch and getting back into condition is a dicier proposition. Trying to do it too fast can actually be dangerous. "Among those at greatest risk for heart-attack death is the habitually sedentary person who engages in unaccustomed physical activity," warns Barry Franklin, physiologist and former chairman of the American Heart Association's Physical Activities Committee. Before starting even a minimal exercise program, therefore, you should call your doctor for a preworkout O.K. or even a checkup.

Once you've been cleared for takeoff, the first step you take may be just that: a walking program that begins modestly and then builds up. Government guidelines recommend at least 30 min. of moderate-intensity activities including walking most days of the week, but Franklin believes in starting even more slowly, if necessary. "I ask my patients if they could manage as little as eight to 10 minutes," he says. "Most of the time they say they can, and then come back having done 14 or 15."

Even that small start can yield big dividends. A good walking program may improve overall physical health as much as 15% in just three months. Since the human body after age 25 experiences, on average, about a 1% falloff in fitness for every additional year of life, "That's a 15-year functional rejuvenation," Franklin says.

For folks aiming for more—weight loss, limberness, a competitive edge in sports—there are other avenues to becoming active again. Depending on how many years you've logged on the couch, high-impact activities such as jogging may not be for you—not if your creaky knees, ankles and hips have anything to say about it. Best to get yourself back in shape with a low-impact activity like swimming, cycling or rowing.

Whatever you choose, begin with a shorter workout than you believe you can handle. "Consciously under-do," advises exercise physiologist Carl Foster of the University of Wisconsin–La Crosse. "We're all 19 behind our eyes, but if you jogged 10 miles a day when you were in college, that doesn't mean you can do it now." Besides, once you're comfortable with a more modest workout

'We're all 19 behind our eyes, but if you jogged 10 miles a day ... in college, that doesn't mean you can do it now.'
—exercise physiologist Carl Foster

load, you can slowly increase it—about 10% a week, Foster recommends. Government guidelines suggest that if you're having trouble finding the time or energy for a full exercise session, you can still get significant health benefits from 30 to 60 min. of exercise broken up into 10- or 15-min. segments throughout the day.

If you're interested in activities that require skill, be willing to bend the rules a little so you can keep up: allow the tennis ball to take an extra bounce, play half-speed hoops on just a portion of the court. Also, don't choose activities that are seasonal, expensive or too solitary: each is a handy excuse for not sticking with your workout program. If you can afford it or if your gym or health club offers it, try to work with a personal trainer at least some of the time, someone who can rein you in when you're doing something wrong, applaud when you're doing something right and, perhaps most important, make you feel guilty if you don't show up at all.

Finally, for all people new to workouts, it pays to continue to play it safe. Be alert for lightheadedness or pain or pressure in the chest. And if you can't speak reasonably comfortably while you're exercising, you're probably getting more winded than is good for you. "The risk from exercise is not too great, but it's there," says Foster. The benefits from doing it right, of course, are enormous. ∎

Exercise Tips for Seniors You may be getting older, but you should still aim to get fit

Being frail or elderly is not an excuse to ignore exercise. If you're over 65, here's how to get started on a fitness regimen.

Check your health If you have high blood pressure or cholesterol, unstable blood-glucose levels or chest pain when walking up stairs, get those symptoms under control before hitting the gym. Update your prescription medications and make sure to take only the drugs you need.

Find a safe workout zone If you choose to exercise at home, make sure it's safe. Keep hallways and other areas well lit and remove loose rugs. Wear proper athletic shoes, not bedroom slippers.

Improve your balance The better your balance, the less likely you are to fall. It may be wise to start with a family member or a trainer to spot you.

Build your strength Strength training is key to long-term independence. Try to target all the major muscles in your trunk, legs and upper body with either free weights or exercise machines. Be sure not to overexert or strain.

Try aerobics Once you've achieved balance and strength, start working on your cardio-vascular system. Walk, bike, swim—do what you enjoy most—choose a heart-pounding exercise you like enough to stick with.

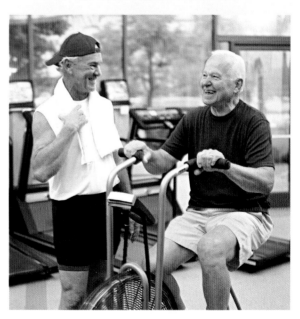

■ On the Horizon Briefs

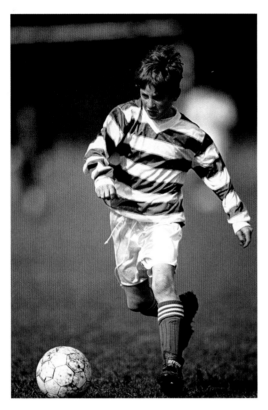

Little Athletes, Big Injuries Train like a pro, strain like a pro

It ought to be hard to take the fun out of play, but if you're an over-eager parent or coach with a young athlete in your charge, you may be guilty of having done so. Weekly sessions of intensive muscle-strengthening, grueling push-up regimens and long intervals on fast-paced treadmills are becoming common for grade-school kids. To sports-medicine professionals, that's a worrying trend. Hard-core training can do kids more harm than good, particularly if they're under 12. Stress fractures in the backs of middle-school football and soccer players have nearly doubled over the past decade as a result of overtraining.

It's young bones that take the worst pounding. Doing the explosive muscle-building movements known as plyometrics can wreak havoc on the skeletal system, especially the epiphyseal, or growth plate, which is essential in bone development, a process that is not complete until the late teens. While our kids certainly do need to exercise more, when injuries start occurring, that's a signal to coaches and parents that they must back off and put the well-being of the child first.

Pumping Up the Workout Here are the latest ways to put fun into getting fit

Fitness gurus keep coming up with inventive ways to work out that promise to be enjoyable and effective for both tenderfeet and old hands. Here are three new techniques that are catching on in U.S. health clubs.

Hooping In classes set to music, exercisers learn a series of Hula Hoop moves that, when combined, work a variety of muscles. "You get the whole body involved," says Rayna McInturf, founder of Los Angeles–based Hoopnotica, the largest adult-size-hoop retailer.
- ■ **Benefits** Hooping makes exercise fun, which means people are more likely to actually do it. It also engages the body's core and helps burn more than 400 calories an hour.
- ■ **Risks** As with any exercise, hooping can be harmful if participants don't stretch properly before working out.
- ■ **Availability** Hooping studios are sprinkled throughout the country, but it can be done anywhere, thanks to the release of two instructional DVDs from Hoopnotica.

Suspension Designed by former Navy SEALS, the Total-body Resistance Exercise (TRX) Suspension Trainer, shown in the picture below, uses heavy-duty nylon webbing, attached to wall brackets, to increase resistance as users perform traditional exercises.
- ■ **Benefits** The TRX works the entire body, engaging the core and working all the supporting muscles.
- ■ **Risks** Users who push themselves too hard invite injuries.
- ■ **Availability** Personal trainers nationwide have adopted the TRX, and many health-club groups are getting onboard.

Fusion Blending yoga and spinning, it makes for a stimulating mind-body workout.
- ■ **Benefits** Cardio-intensive cycling followed by flexibility-increasing yoga helps stretch and condition muscles.
- ■ **Risks** Switching activities too quickly can lead to injury.
- ■ **Availability** Starting to catch on nationally. Ask your gym!

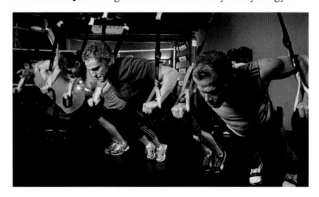

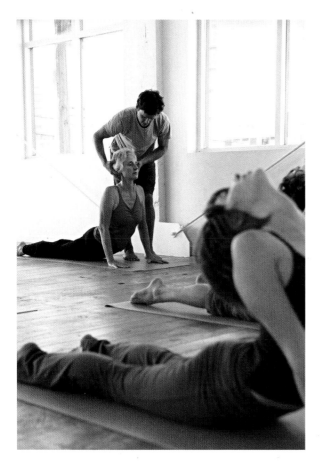

The Perils of Yoga As injuries rise, it's time to get back to the basics

Bad-mouthing yoga seems like begging for a hit of evil karma. But with more than 14 million people practicing yoga or Tai Chi nationwide, up 136% since 2000, health professionals across the country are dealing with the increasing fallout from yoga gone awry. Over the past three years, 13,000 Americans were treated in an emergency room or a doctor's office for yoga-related injuries such as muscle strains or back-aches, according to the Consumer Product Safety Commission. Experts say most of these injuries are sustained by "weekend warrior" baby boomers who begin yoga without realizing that their bodies are no longer what they used to be.

The truth is, yoga does not offer a comprehensive way to get fit, though it does help reduce stress. It's not the best way to lose weight either. A typical 50-min. class of hatha yoga burns off fewer calories than are contained in three Oreos—about the same as a slow, 50-min. walk. Part of the problem is ill-trained instructors who forget that yoga is intended to be an exercise that trains mind, body and spirit together—it is not a shortcut to fitness.

Alcohol and Exercise Working as a team, they may help your health

If you want to live a long and healthy life, you're probably trying to eat right, exercise regularly and get enough sleep. Good steps. Now how about adding a little alcohol to your regimen?

That's right. It is well documented that tossing back a few drinks in a week (and that means a few: up to one a day for women, up to two for men) has potential heart benefits. But researchers in Denmark decided to look further. Could drinking alcohol have a benefit similar to that of exercise?

"If you don't want to exercise too much," asks Dr. Morten Gronbaek, epidemiologist with Denmark's National Institute of Public Health, "can you trade it for one to two drinks per day and be fine?" A study Gronbaek and colleagues published in 2008 in the *European Heart Journal* suggests the answer just may be yes. Surveying 12,000 people over a 20-year period, they found that exercise and drinking alcohol each had an independent beneficial effect on the heart and a compounded effect when practiced together.

People who don't drink at all and don't exercise had the highest risk of heart disease in the study. People who drink moderately and also exercise had a 50% lower risk. Teetotaling exercisers had a 30% decreased risk, as did moderately drinking couch potatoes. "There's an additional protective effect to doing both," Gronbaek told TIME. "That's the new finding."

Why is a drink beneficial? Alcohol and exercise affect your heart health in similar ways, increasing good cholesterol, or HDL (high-density lipoproteins), and cleaning the circulatory system's pipes.

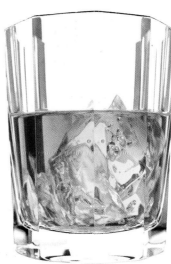

Three caveats: stick to the rules of one drink a day for women and up to two drinks a day for men. The regimen only helps those age 45 and older (sorry, twentysomethings). And it goes without saying that you should never drink your weekly allotment all at once.

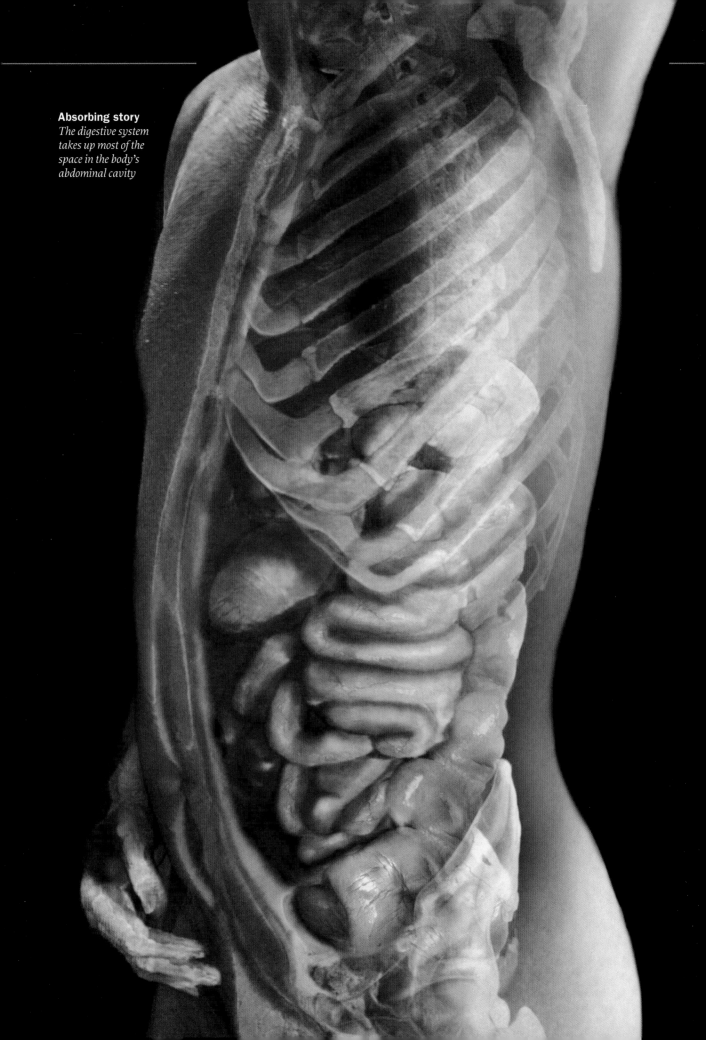

Absorbing story
The digestive system takes up most of the space in the body's abdominal cavity

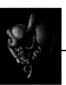

Power Supply

You are what you eat, eventually: the digestive system

PICTURE YOURSELF WITH A POCKET FULL OF $100 bills, trapped in an arcade filled with vending machines that offer tantalizing goods but accept only quarters, and you'll have some idea of the vital work your digestive system performs. Your body cannot use the proteins, fats and carbohydrates in the way they arrive—as large, complex molecules—in the food we eat. What every cell in your body does crave, however, is small amino acids, fatty acids and simple sugars—the more refined, delicately diced versions of these compounds—along with salt, a handful of other minerals and some vitamins. Your digestive system is the nutrient currency exchanger, responsible for converting the large nutrient bills you start with into smaller and smaller units, until you finally end up with the pennies you need.

But this doesn't happen all at once—or in one place. Your digestive system is essentially a single long tube, consisting of hollow organs that are connected to one another. They begin with your mouth, where food enters the body, is chewed into smaller pieces, then is swallowed and sent through the esophagus to the stomach. The next organs are the large and small intestines, followed by the rectum and anus, where digested food waste leaves the body. The digestive organs are lined by the mucosa, a wall of tiny glands that make both protective mucus, juices that help break down food, and hormones. (Spent layers of mucosa constantly peel away from the inside of the digestive tract and pass out of the body as waste.) Beneath the mucosa lies a layer of smooth, involuntary muscle that pushes and squeezes food along the length of the tube, crushing, mashing and mixing it with digestive juices.

From mouth to anus, your digestive tract is between five and six times your height—almost 40 ft. in some tall adults. The time needed for food to journey through the tube is as much as 36 hr. In a single day, the digestive tract typically secretes about 3 gal. of chemicals that aid in digestion, including more than 1.5 qt. of saliva and another 1.5 qt. of juices from the pancreas. In the course of an average lifetime, the human digestive tract will process more than 30 tons of food.

Alongside the tube are a trio of organs that aren't hollow and only secrete substances onto food. The liver makes bile, an important digestive juice that is stored in the gall bladder, while the pancreas makes insulin, a hormone that regulates blood sugar levels. The pancreas also makes enzymes that help break down carbohydrates and digest some fats and oils, and it manufactures pancreatic juice, an alkaline natural antacid that neutralizes the dangerously acidic contents of the stomach as they pass into the small intestine, rendering them harmless.

Human digestion depends upon the action of dozens of separate enzymes, each of which is specialized to con-

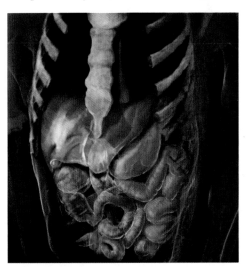

Inner tubes *Major organs of the digestive system include the esophagus, liver, pancreas, stomach and large and small intestines*

vert a single substance, such as cleaving large proteins into smaller, simpler models or altering sucrose (table sugar) into glucose and fructose, more manageable sugars that can be absorbed directly into the bloodstream.

When the body's chemical change machines have completed their work, proteins, carbohydrates and fats —the high-denomination molecules that, along with water, make up most food—are reduced to their simplest, smallest and most useful parts. But as with the dollars that seem to fill our wallets so briefly, it won't be long until our tummy reminds us it's time for a refill. ∎

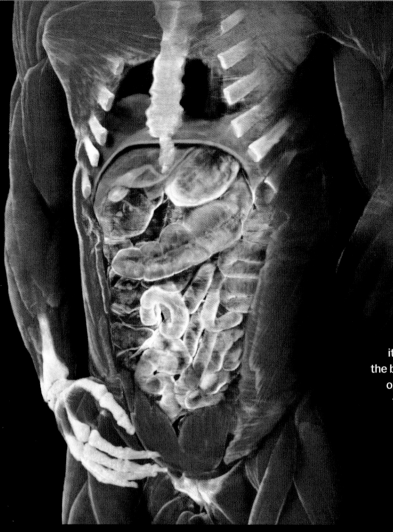

Alimentary canal *Numerous organs combine to digest and absorb food, including the mouth, esophagus, stomach and intestines. Stomach acids that help dissolve food are so strong that they burn away the organ's protective mucous lining, which must replace 50 million cells every few seconds. This gastric mucosa completely replenishes itself every three days*

■ Anatomy Lesson
The Digestive System

Human digestion is an assembly-line process— actually, a disassembly-line process—that consists of six basic kinds of work. It begins with *ingestion,* the act of putting food into your mouth. In *mechanical digestion,* we break down food by chewing it. Then enzymes and acids perform *chemical digestion*, while *movement* involves pushing food from one station to another, such as from the mouth to the stomach. *Absorption* is the payoff: food that has been converted into the kind of molecules that fuel every cell in your body is transferred into the bloodstream, for transport. Finally, in *elimination,* digestive waste passes out of your body, through defecation.

Mechanical and chemical digestion both start in the mouth: while the teeth mash food into a compact ball called a bolus, enzymes known as amylases begin dissolving and simplifying starches, turning them into sugars. Once you swallow, digestive movement begins, and it continues with a series of involuntary muscle contractions called peristalsis. As food passes into the esophagus (the 10-in. tube connecting the mouth to the stomach), a ring of muscle in front of the bolus relaxes, allowing it to fall. At the same time, a ring of muscle behind the bolus contracts, pushing it downward. This opening-and-closing peristaltic wave continues in the stomach—where its action can sometimes be heard as "grumbling"—and in the intestines.

Chemical digestion begins once food hits the stomach. Here, acids so strong and caustic that they would kill you if they escaped your stomach further decompose food into its chemical building blocks. The stomach also begins absorbing food in a minor way: water, alcohol and some drugs are transferred into the bloodstream here, but little else is allowed entry.

By the time food leaves the stomach, the boluses that entered from the esophagus are transformed into a pastelike slurry called chyme, which then passes to the small intestine. Here, chemical digestion continues, now aided by enzymes from the liver, gall bladder and pancreas, which transform large proteins into amino acids, carbohydrates and sugars into glucose, and fats into fatty acids. But the small intestine's real specialty is absorption: millions of fingerlike projections, the villi, absorb these nutrients (as well as others, such as mineral irons, vitamins and some forms of digested fat) and pass them off to microscopic blood vessels, which carry them throughout the body to hungry cellular consumers.

When the small intestine has completed breaking down and absorbing chyme, what is passed onto the large intestine, or colon, consists mostly of fiber (which is never digested) and waste chemicals. This dried-out remnant matter, or feces, is about one-third the size and weight of the food originally ingested. In a final push of peristaltic contraction, our body excretes this waste matter through the anus.

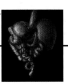

Common Digestive Diseases and Disorders

Gastritis Several conditions whose defining symptom is inflammation of the stomach lining; most often caused by excessive alcohol consumption, prolonged use of nonsteroidal anti-inflammatory drugs (NSAIDs) such as aspirin or ibuprofen or infection with bacteria such as *Helicobacter pylori (H. pylori)*, a common bacteria. Can develop after major surgery, injury, burns or severe infections.

■ **Symptoms** *Abdominal upset or pain; belching, bloating, nausea, vomiting; blood in vomit; black stools.*

■ **Treatment** Drugs to reduce stomach acid; avoidance of specific foods.

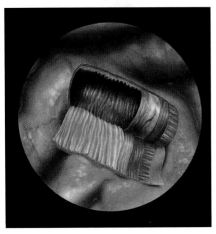

Intestinal wall *This illustration shows the lining of the lower intestine; peptic ulcers appear here and in the stomach*

Heartburn Also called acid reflux; occurs when the lower esophageal sphincter opens spontaneously, for varying periods of time, or does not close properly and stomach contents rise up into the esophagus, bringing with them acidic digestive juices.

■ **Symptoms** *Burning pain in the lower chest or mid-abdomen. In most children and some adults, also signalled by a dry cough, shortness of breath or trouble swallowing.*

■ **Treatment** Smoking cessation and diet modification; medications including antacids, foaming agents, H2 blockers, proton pump inhibitors or prokinetics; fundoplication surgery, in which the upper part of the stomach is wrapped around the lower esophageal sphincter to prevent acid reflux.

Irritable Bowel Syndrome A functional disorder rather than a disease, IBS is a group of symptoms involving extra sensitivity in the nerves and muscles in the colon. Although painful, IBS does not damage the colon or larger digestive system.

■ **Symptoms** *Abdominal pain or discomfort, often with cramping, bloating, gas, diarrhea or constipation.*

■ **Treatment** Diet modification; laxatives, antispasmodics or antidepressants; stress relief.

Pancreatitis An inflammation of the pancreas, either of short duration (acute) or long-lasting (chronic), in which digestive enzymes intended for the small intestine instead become active inside the pancreas, where they start "digesting" the organ itself.

■ **Symptoms** *Often begins with pain in the upper abdomen, especially during and after meals; swollen and tender abdomen; nausea; fever; and rapid pulse. For chronic pancreatitis, symptoms include nausea, vomiting, weight loss and fatty stools.*

■ **Treatment** Acute pancreatitis often improves on its own. For chronic cases: a diet high in carbohydrates and low in fat; pancreatic enzymes may be prescribed; surgery to relieve pain, drain an enlarged pancreatic duct or remove part of the pancreas.

Peptic Ulcers Also called stomach ulcers; sores on the lining of the stomach or duodenum (the beginning of the small intestine), believed to be caused most often by *H. pylori*. Some ulcers are also caused by long-term use of NSAIDS, like aspirin and ibuprofen; in a few cases, cancerous tumors in the stomach or pancreas cause ulcers.

■ **Symptoms** *Most often, abdominal discomfort that comes and goes for several days or weeks (often a few hours after a meal or in the middle of the night). Other symptoms: weight loss, poor appetite, nausea, vomiting.*

■ **Treatment** Most peptic ulcers are easily cured with antibiotics that kill *H. pylori*, reduce stomach acid and protect the stomach lining. Acid-suppressing drugs may also be used.

Source: National Institutes of Health

Digestive System Terms to Know

Bile Secretions of the liver that aid in digestion and absorption and stimulate coordinated contractions in the intestinal tract, or peristalsis.

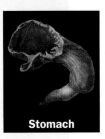

Stomach

Borborygmi Rumbling abdominal sounds due to gas gurgling with liquid as it passes through the intestines.

Enteric nervous system Part of the autonomic nervous system within the walls of the digestive tract. The ENS regulates digestion and the muscle contractions that eliminate solid waste.

Gastrointestinal tract Or GI; it is the muscular tube that runs from the mouth to the anus; also called the alimentary canal or digestive tract.

H2 blockers Medicines that reduce the amount of acid produced by the stomach.

Proton pump inhibitor Or PPI; a drug that limits acid secretion in the stomach.

Villi Small, tubelike projections in the walls of the small intestine that absorb nutrients.

Source: National Institutes of Health

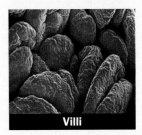

Villi

■On the Horizon Briefs

Burning Questions Peptic ulcers are no longer a mystery, and cures are close at hand

It has been nearly 25 years since Drs. Barry Marshall and J. Robin Warren showed that the vast majority of peptic ulcers are caused by a bacterium called *Helicobacter pylori,* a discovery that earned the pair a Nobel Prize in 2005. Yet a surprising number of ulcer sufferers still don't realize that their stomach pains can easily and effectively be cured with antibiotics.

A peptic ulcer is a sore in the protective lining of the stomach or duodenum (the upper part of the small intestine). The most common symptom is a burning pain between your belly button and your breastbone. It's usually worse at night or when your stomach is empty.

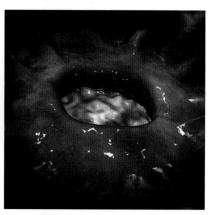

No one knows exactly how *H. pylori* gets into the stomach—it may be via eating, touching or even kissing—and 80% of people who are infected with the bug never develop ulcers. There may even be some truth to the old myths: that stress and spicy food don't create ulcers, but they can certainly make them worse.

Some ulcers, however, can't be pinned on *H. pylori.* Instead, they are caused by prescription and over-the-counter anti-inflammatory drugs, such as ibuprofen, aspirin and naproxen, that interfere with the body's mechanism for protecting the stomach lining. The ulcers are particularly common among the elderly, who take a lot of those medicines. The ulcers begin to heal as soon as they stop taking the drugs.

Ulcers caused by *H. pylori* can take longer to heal—from two to six weeks. The usual treatment is a combination of antibiotics, acid suppressors and something to protect the stomach lining. Bleeding ulcers that eat all the way through the stomach lining are a serious medical condition that can be life threatening. If you find yourself experiencing sharp, sudden pain in the upper abdomen or have black or bloody stools or vomiting, don't wait: get emergency care.

Eat Your Germs Probiotic foods are a hit with consumers. Are they right for you?

With the enormous success of its yogurt line named Activia, which is fortified with extra, good-for-you bacteria, the Dannon Co. seems to have kick-started a new food trend, called probiotics. Other companies are coming forward with probiotic yogurt drinks and fortified beverages, which are also finding a market. The good news: there is a fair body of science suggesting that it makes sense to choose these foods. In the digestive tract, the "superstar" bacteria help regulate and restore peristalsis, the rhythmic motion of the intestine that pushes digested food through, aiding regularity.

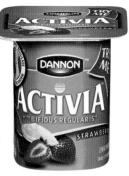

Not everyone is sold, however; the U.S. Food and Drug Administration (FDA) is relatively neutral on the subject, and those with weakened immune systems or who are critically ill would be well advised to stay away from eating live bacteria.

The Raw Deal Should you be getting your milk straight from the cow?

Since 1987, the FDA has required that milk sold between states for human consumption be pasteurized, meaning it must first be heated to kill off most of the bacteria that might be lurking in the barn or flourishing in the cow. But a growing number of natural-food fans are demanding the right to bring milk from teat to table, convinced that pasteurization strips away the very stuff that makes milk nutritious to begin with. Farmers are more than willing to meet the demand, since raw-milk products command a thick price premium.

Fans argue that heating destroys the good bacteria—the same probiotic critters found in Activia yogurt—as well as enzymes that can aid your health. Food-safety authorities

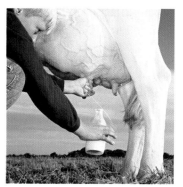

warn of a potential uptick in the milk-borne illnesses that pasteurization was designed to prevent.

Who's right? For now, the available evidence suggests that without a bug-killing step like pasteurization, even the cleanest dairy cannot always expect to produce safe raw milk.

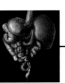

Welcome the Probe
Smoke and drink? A timely colonoscopy may save your life

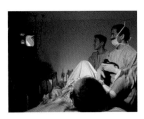

It's never easy to convince people it's a good idea to get their colon probed from the inside by a 5-ft.-long tube, but it's never been more important for some of us to grin and, uh, bare it. A 2006 study of more than 160,000 colon-cancer patients published in the *Archives of Internal Medicine* found that the cancers of patients who smoked tobacco or drank alcohol, both of which increase risk of the disease, were diagnosed an average of 5.2 years earlier than were those of other patients.

The clear implication is that smokers and drinkers should be getting screened earlier than ever for colorectal cancer. Doctors usually recommend that patients schedule their first exam on or near their 50th birthday. If you get a colonoscopy—considered the gold standard of screenings because it allows doctors to examine the whole length of the lower intestine and snip off any precancerous polyps they find at the same time—you may not need to be screened again for 10 years. If you use one of the less definitive tests— a flexible sigmoidoscopy, barium enema or simple stool analysis—you should get tested more frequently. Why? Because colorectal cancer remains one of the top three causes of cancer deaths in the U.S. (after lung and breast cancer), but it doesn't have to be; 90% of cases detected early can be cured.

'Having a colonoscopy is a heck of a lot easier than facing a diagnosis of colon cancer.'
—Katie Couric

Nobody, including colonoscopy advocate and CBS news anchor Katie Couric, whose husband died of the disease, likes to talk about getting their backside probed, but, as she told TIME Health columnist Sanjay Gupta, M.D., "Fear and embarrassment are major obstacles, but educated, well-informed people who want to have long lives should force themselves to get over those feelings. The time to be screened for colon cancer is when you are feeling well and not having symptoms. Having a colonoscopy is a heck of a lot easier than facing a diagnosis of colon cancer."

Meanwhile, there are plenty of steps all of us can take to improve our odds of avoiding colon cancer. Exercise is good for both our hearts and our colons. We should also try to eat less red meat (which stresses the digestive system) and more vegetables, fruit and—above all—fiber. There's no reason to become a victim of a disease that you can beat thanks to an early warning.

Liver The body's largest organ is a critical multi-tasker

The liver is the utility infielder of the body, performing essential—if far from glamorous—functions that keep us humming along. Without the liver, our circulatory, digestive, immune and endocrine systems couldn't do their jobs. Weighing some 3 lbs. in the average adult, this two-lobed organ lies just below the heart on the right side of the upper abdomen. From this perch it creates, filters and stores key substances from bile to sugars.

The liver produces bile, an alkaline compound that helps the body break down fats for absorption. Connected to the bloodstream via the hepatic duct, it also churns out cholesterol and triglyceride fats, which, despite their bad reputation, are essential to maintaining the elasticity of the circulatory system. In fetuses, it stands in for undeveloped bone marrow, helping to produce red blood cells. The liver also produces clotting agents for the blood, as well as albumin, a component of blood serum.

As a storehouse, the liver is a repository for glucose, vitamin B_{12} and minerals. As a filter, it removes antigens, important to the body's immune system. As a regulator of metabolism, it helps moderate our level of sugars, as well as of insulin and other hormones. Finally, the liver is also a conversion center, where ammonia is transformed into urea, and sugars are converted into forms the body can use for energy.

Utility player *The twin-lobed liver sits on top of the gall bladder, yellow. The hepatic portal vein, bottom right, carries blood to the liver*

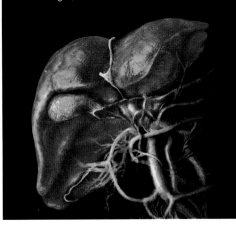

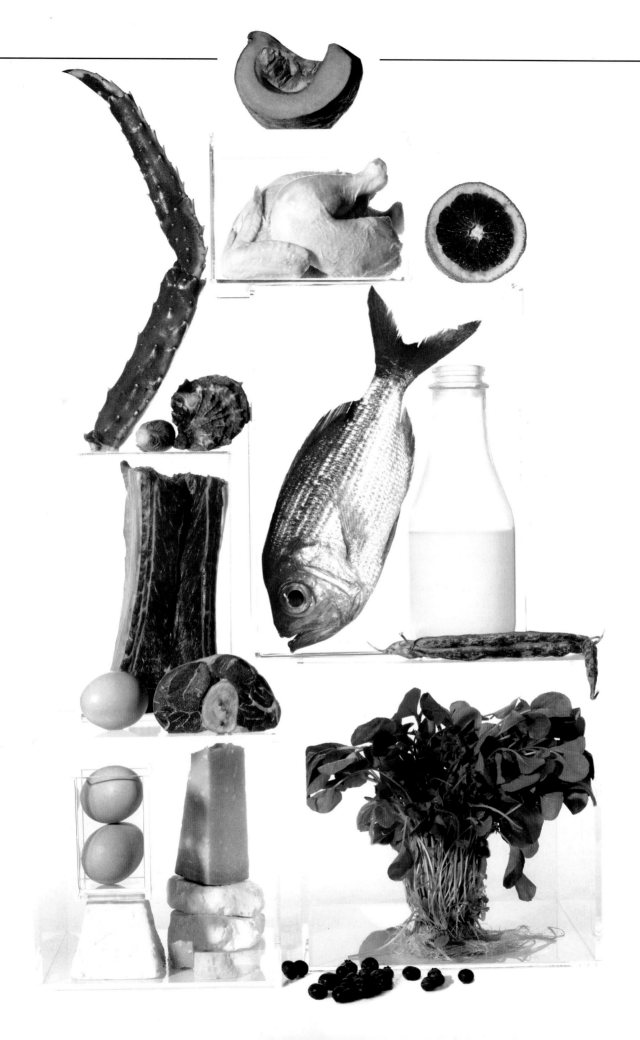

The Science of Appetite

Discovering what drives us to eat may help us control the urge

HUMAN BEINGS HAVE ALWAYS HAD A COMPLICATED relationship with food. Staying alive from day to day requires our bodies to keep a lot of systems running just so, but most of them—circulatory, respiratory, endocrine—operate without our having to give them a second thought. Eating is different. Like sex, it's a voluntary thing. And like sex, it's a sine qua non to keep the species going. So nature rigs the game, making sure we pursue them both by making sure we can't resist them. In the case of food, that can spell trouble. Nature never planned for what could happen when unchecked appetites were suddenly matched by unchecked resources. But we're seeing it now.

Postindustrial humans—as any trip to an all-you-can-eat buffet will tell you—have become a soft, sedentary, overfed lot. It's not just that 67% of the U.S. population is either overweight or obese (including about 17% of children ages 12 to 19); it's that we know that fact full well and seem helpless to control ourselves. We lose weight and routinely regain it; we vow to eat healthfully and almost always lapse. Our doctors warn us about our rising blood pressure and creeping cholesterol, and we get briefly spooked—until we're offered the next helping of cheesecake or curly fries, our appetite shouts down our reason and we're at it again.

Just why is our appetite so powerful a driver of our behavior, and, more important, how can we bring it to heel? If that question has long defied easy answers, it's no wonder. Understanding all the aspects of a process as complex as appetite—one that involves taste, smell, sight, texture, brain chemistry, gut chemistry, metabolism and, most confounding of all, psychology—is very difficult. But as scientists probe the brain, the stomach and the substances that link them, they're solving the puzzle of appetite. The solution may begin with a substance that is often called the hunger hormone, ghrelin.

First identified in 1999, ghrelin is produced in the gut in response to the body's regular meal schedules—and, according to some theories, the mere sight or smell of food—and is designed to give rise to the empty feeling we recognize as the desire to eat. When ghrelin hits the brain, it heads straight for three areas: the hindbrain, which controls the body's automatic, unconscious processes; the hypothalamus, which governs metabolism; and the mesolimbic reward center in the midbrain, where feelings of pleasure and satisfaction are processed. That's a neural triple play that guarantees that when ghrelin talks, the brain will listen.

Humans are creatures of dietary habit; our appetites follow the clock. Dr. David Cummings, an associate professor of medicine at the University of Washington,

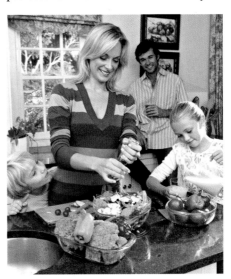

Slim chance *Eating larger portions of salad and smaller portions of fatty foods is a simple way to control appetites*

has conducted studies in which he measured ghrelin levels in people's blood every 20 min. and found that they reliably spike as mealtimes approach. Add or subtract a daily meal, and you soon gain or lose a surge.

One of the reasons gastric-bypass surgery can work in severely obese people—apart from the fact that it reduces the carrying capacity of the stomach—is that it also appears to turn down the ghrelin spigot. An Italian study even looked at ghrelin in anorexics and found that levels of the hormone were chronically high—a chemical alarm that the self-starvers trained themselves to ignore. This research confirmed ghrelin's role in driving appetite, both when we really need to eat and when we merely expect to.

If ghrelin were all there was to it, we would happily eat ourselves to death. But even as one system is gunning our hunger higher, another is standing by to slow things down. Scientists have now identified several substances that travel northward from the gut to signal that the stomach is full and suppress appetite. The first is a peptide released by the upper intestine called cholecystokinin (CCK), which sends a fleeting mes-

'It's not big portions that make you eat more. It's big portions of calories.'

sage of satiety to the brain. But it's the two hormones that follow, GLP-1 and PYY, that really slam on the brakes: they not only tell your brain you've had enough but also tell your stomach not to move more food into the intestines, where the real business of digestion takes place, until what's there has been broken down some.

The body has one other, bigger weapon it can roll out: leptin. An appetite-suppressing hormone discovered in 1994, leptin is produced by body fat itself, usually in direct proportion to how much of the tissue you're carrying. The fatter you are, the more leptin you produce. The result should be that fatter people want to eat less. But at some point the stuff simply stops working—or at least stops keeping pace with the numbers on the scale—and the desire to eat overrides leptin's signal to stop.

As scientists probe the drivers of appetite, the goal is to rejigger the body's systems and bring them under control. Some researchers are looking deeper into the brain, studying the receptor sites on individual neurons to which appetite-control chemicals bond, in

hopes of discovering why the signals sent by leptin aren't tracking. Some are exploring genetic mutations that also retard leptin's impact. Others are examining the pace of the body's operating systems, seeking drugs that will boost metabolism and make overeaters more efficient at burning their calorie intake.

Some researchers are even exploring a surprising link between excessive eating and the patterns of drug addiction. Most chronic consumers of both food and drugs are aware that their habits can kill them, yet few have the power to stop. In both kinds of people, there is a general deficit of activity in the brain's mesolimbic region, which suggests that the compulsive intake of food or chemicals may be an attempt to compensate for this shortfall. The goal is to develop a drug that will regulate this activity.

But if you're trying to get your appetite under control today, waiting for a breakthrough drug won't help. Barbara Rolls, a professor of nutritional sciences at Pennsylvania State University, advocates one sound way to attack hunger even more aggressively. In a best-selling 2007 book, she advocates what she calls a "volumetrics" eating plan—the kind of prefab word that cries out diet fad but in this case describes a sensible idea, if followed in moderation. Her advice: Consume foods that are high in volume but not in calories in order to stimulate the digestive system's distension nerves, another signal to stop eating. It's the difference between, say, a large, filling salad with a low-calorie load and a small, unfilling brownie with a high one.

"This whole idea of eating smaller portions—I'm really fed up with it," Rolls says. "It's not big portions that make you eat more. It's big portions of calories. If you eat big portions of fruits and vegetables, they displace other foods." If the human brain could invent the supermarket and food court, it seems it must be able to develop ways to control how we use them. ∎

The Decision

1. PANGS

Role Hunger isn't just in your head. When your stomach is empty, it contracts, sending signals along the vagus nerve to the brain

Effect Hunger affects both voluntary and involuntary physical systems. You can ignore the contractions, but a host of other signals will soon take over

2. SENSES

Role The smell and sight of food can stimulate appetite. Your body also wants a variety of sensations, which is one reason you want dessert after a steak

Effect Closing your eyes or walking away may help, but only temporarily. Your body knows when you typically eat and you'll get hungry at those times each day

LOOKS GOOD

3. GHRELIN

Role This hormone, produced in the stomach, sends strong feelings of hunger to the brain. It's rising ghrelin concentrations that account for hunger as mealtimes approach

Effect The more ghrelin, the more hunger you feel. Gastric-bypass surgery reduces ghrelin production, helping obese patients feel full longer

EAT!

4. STRETCHING

Role As you eat, your stomach and intestines begin to stretch, sending nerve impulses to the brain that quiet appetite

Effect It's a slow process. Your stomach may say stop eating, but your brain won't hear the message for several more minutes

Evolution has programmed us to eat as much as we can, whenever we can. Breaking that cycle means thwarting overlapping systems that try to keep you fat. The key players:

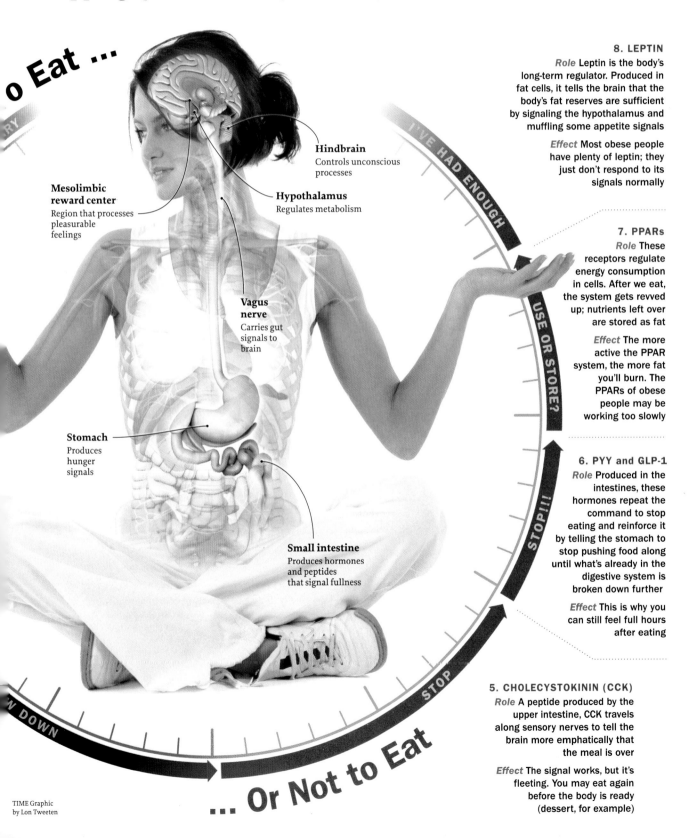

o Eat ...

Mesolimbic reward center
Region that processes pleasurable feelings

Hindbrain
Controls unconscious processes

Hypothalamus
Regulates metabolism

Vagus nerve
Carries gut signals to brain

Stomach
Produces hunger signals

Small intestine
Produces hormones and peptides that signal fullness

I'VE HAD ENOUGH

USE OR STORE?

STOP!!!

STOP

N DOWN

... Or Not to Eat

8. LEPTIN
Role Leptin is the body's long-term regulator. Produced in fat cells, it tells the brain that the body's fat reserves are sufficient by signaling the hypothalamus and muffling some appetite signals

Effect Most obese people have plenty of leptin; they just don't respond to its signals normally

7. PPARs
Role These receptors regulate energy consumption in cells. After we eat, the system gets revved up; nutrients left over are stored as fat

Effect The more active the PPAR system, the more fat you'll burn. The PPARs of obese people may be working too slowly

6. PYY and GLP-1
Role Produced in the intestines, these hormones repeat the command to stop eating and reinforce it by telling the stomach to stop pushing food along until what's already in the digestive system is broken down further

Effect This is why you can still feel full hours after eating

5. CHOLECYSTOKININ (CCK)
Role A peptide produced by the upper intestine, CCK travels along sensory nerves to tell the brain more emphatically that the meal is over

Effect The signal works, but it's fleeting. You may eat again before the body is ready (dessert, for example)

TIME Graphic
by Lon Tweeten

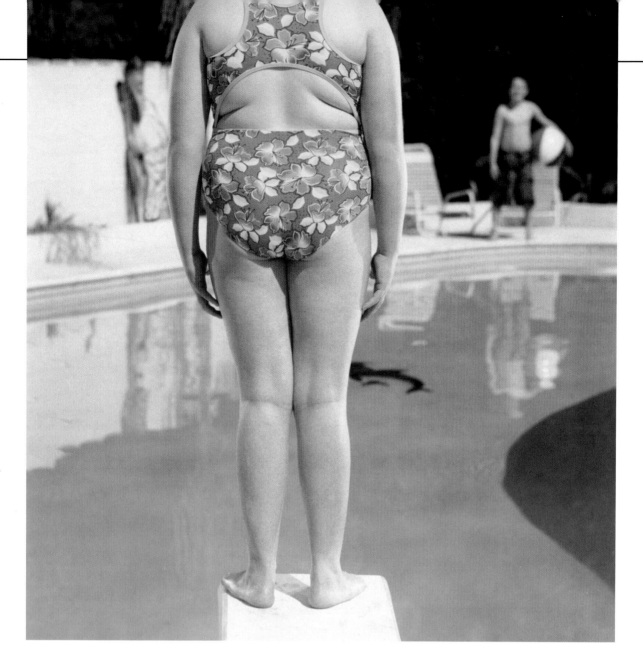

Today's Kids: Living Large

How to turn around America's epidemic of early obesity

HIGH CHOLESTEROL. SOARING BLOOD PRESSURE. A FATTY liver. Dangerously high insulin levels. Even a first-year medical student could recognize the signs of a middle-aged patient struggling with weight problems and diabetes and probably heading for a heart attack.

And in most cases, that med student would be right. But increasingly, the same deadly mix of problems is appearing in a startlingly younger population: teens and adolescents barely through their second decade of life. In 1971 only 4% of 6-to-11-year-old kids were obese; by 2004, the figure had leaped to 18.8%. And that's just obesity. Include all overweight kids, and a whopping 32% of all American children now carry more pounds than they should. It gets worse: a staggering 90% of overweight

kids already have at least one avoidable risk factor for heart disease, such as high cholesterol or hypertension. Type 2 diabetes is being diagnosed in teens as young as 15. Health experts warn that the current generation of children may be the first in American history to have a shorter life expectancy than their parents do.

It's hardly a secret how American children have come to this unhealthy state. In the era of the 64-oz. soda, the 1,200-calorie burger and the pizza buffet as an everyday choice in many school cafeterias, food companies produce enough food for every American to consume a belt-popping 3,800 calories per day, even though an adult needs only 2,350 to survive and children need even fewer.

Yet not only are kids consuming far more calories than

they can possibly use, but they're also doing less and less with them. The transformation of American homes into high-def, Web-enabled, TiVo-equipped entertainment centers means that children who come home after a largely sedentary day at a school desk spend an average of three more sedentary hours in front of some kind of screen. Schools have contributed, with shrinking budgets causing more and more of them to slash physical-education programs. Today, 25% or fewer of all school-aged kids participate in phys-ed programs. Other factors are important too: income, race, education and, in particular, heredity, all play a role in the propensity toward obesity.

What can parents do? Children should eat five or more servings of fruits and veggies daily. They should be eating a healthy breakfast, which can fill them up and make them less likely to snack on nutrition-free but high-calorie foods. They should be getting at least one hour of moderate physical activity each day. They should be spending fewer than two hours in front of a TV or computer screen each day.

Or rather, the entire family should be doing these things—together. In fact, you can boil down all the experts' messages on childhood obesity to simply being a good role model. As parents, we need to think about how our eating and exercising behaviors are perceived by our kids. If parents become more active and committed to eating a healthy diet, children will do the same.

And there are flickers of hope. In May 2008, epidemiologists were encouraged when the *Journal of the American Medical Association* published a study of 8,165 children showing that for the first time in decades the increase in U.S. childhood obesity had leveled off. It's not certain if the plateau is a sign that public-awareness programs and improved menus in many school cafeterias are yielding results or simply that some kind of saturation point has been reached, with most kids who are genetically susceptible to gaining too much weight having already done so.

One thing is clear: the battle against child obesity will be a long, multifront war. Parents are fighting it in the home as they learn how to make healthier meals available to their families, set better examples with their own food choices and manage the critical issues of self-esteem that can be so disabling for overweight kids. And teachers, mentors and public role models are fighting it in the schools and in the community as they help kids navigate a culture that fosters fat but idealizes thin. Ultimately, the lesson these children are learning is that they should live as fit as their body type and genes allow—and then reap the healthy rewards. ■

10 Tips to Get Your Kids Moving

1. Pull the Plug TV, video games and the Internet seem to have an unbreakable hold on young people. But parents need to be parents. Set limits for screen time and make physical activity mandatory.

2. Walk This Way Walking is the best way to begin a fitness program. Wherever kids live, you can find places to stride and stairs to climb. Get moving!

3. Stay Flexible A routine can be a boon for discipline, but don't be too strict. Schedule longer activities for days with free time. Plan fitness dates with friends.

4. Game Your Play Fitness is easier when it's fun, and why limit yourself to traditional sports? The more active games of Nintendo's Wii system or improvised outdoor games are fine.

5. Make It a Contest Challenge friends and family members to imaginative fitness contests. Start slow but build up; keep it creative—and be sure to have fun.

6. Mighty Milers Running is a great way for kids to boost their confidence while getting fit, and it can be a great social experience too. Most towns have "fun runs" that are open to all ages.

7. Spin Your Wheels Forget the car and move by other means. Get kids rolling on bikes, scooters or skates.

8. You Know You Can Dance Can the inhibition, crank up the music and shake, bounce and move it. Pick a style, fake it or make one up. Yes, air guitar counts.

9. Take a Hike Organize outings on weekends; even a long walk in the park will do. Bring a ball or Frisbee.

10. Start Young Get kids going with tag or hide-and-seek. Ask tiny tots to run like a gorilla or hop like a bunny.

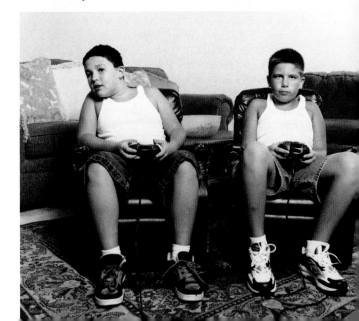

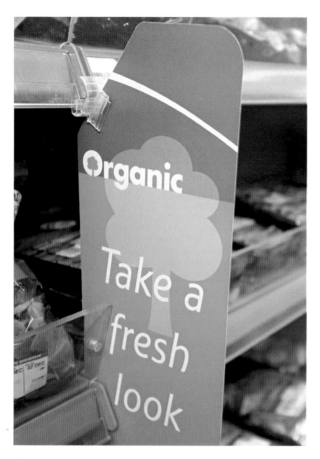

Organic Food Is it better for you—or merely a pricey fad?

Are there real health benefits to eating organic food? If so, are some organic fruits and vegetables better than others? And how do you choose? First of all, scientists have yet to document a definite, long-term negative effect of modern pesticides on our bodies, so while organic foods do you no harm, they may not turn out to be as beneficial as you think.

To date, most studies have found either no difference between organic and conventional produce or very small pluses in the organic column. However, when researchers at the University of California at Davis compared levels of two antioxidants—quercetin and kaempferol—in tomatoes, they found that those grown in organic fields yielded significantly higher amounts of these nutrients than their conventional counterparts.

Quercetin and kaempferol are flavonoids, which are associated with reduced risk of heart disease, certain cancers and even some forms of dementia. The team also found that the greater the number of seasons tomatoes are grown in organic fields, the higher the level of the flavonoids. More research to quantify any benefits of eating organic is under way. For now, the best advice is simple: eat more fruits and veggies, whatever the label reads.

A New Diet Equation Choose the diet that fits your shape

New research indicates that the places on your body where you pack on extra pounds may provide a clue to determining which diet works best for you. The key is insulin, which triggers the way the body stores excess fat. In a study of 73 obese adults published in 2007 in the *Journal of the American Medical Association,* researchers looked at high- and low-insulin secretors. It was already known that people who rapidly secrete a lot of insulin after eating a little bit of sugar tend to carry their excess weight around their waist—the so-called apple shape. People who secrete less insulin carry their excess fat around their hips—the pear shape.

The study found that high-insulin, apple-shaped people will not lose as much weight on a diet that restricts fat calories as they will on a low-glycemic-load diet—one that restricts simple carbohydrates from sugary and starchy foods like cookies and potatoes. Low-secreting, pear-shaped people, however, will do equally well on either type of diet.

We've listed at right the principles of the three most popular diets in the U.S. Another 2007 study found that regardless of body shape, the Atkins diet produces the greatest short-term weight loss. However, Atkins adherents tend to fall off the low-carb wagon and quickly gain back unwanted pounds. What's clear from the first study is that apple-shaped people should probably not choose low-fat diets, but it didn't clarify if the Ornish-style vegetarian diet works better for them. As for the pear-shaped, it remains a toss-up. But it can't hurt them to follow the most basic dieting advice around: eat less.

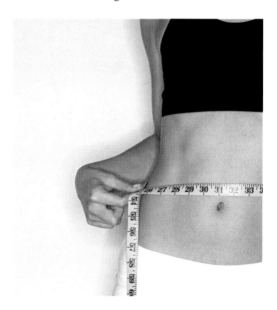

Three Diets A look at how they stack up

Here are America's three most popular diets, noting what you can eat, what they do to your body and why they can end up letting you down.

■ The Atkins Diet

Philosophy Cut carbohydrates—they make you hungrier. Load up on fats and proteins like meat.

How It Works When the body takes in very few carbs, it gets its energy by burning fat rather than carbs, as the liver turns stored fat into chemicals called ketones, which are used for fuel (and can give you less-than-fresh breath).

Downside Long-term adherence. It's hard to stick to a diet that restricts such a big chunk of the food pyramid.

■ Weight Watchers Diet

Philosophy Portion control. Nothing is off-limits, but everything must be in moderation.

How It Works Smaller portions mean fewer calories are taken in, so less fat gets stored. A point system helps tabulate and limit daily consumption. To lose a pound a week, you may need to consume 500 fewer calories a day.

Downside Hunger. Small portions can leave stomachs growling.

■ The Ornish Diet

Philosophy Kiss meat goodbye. Cut down on fats and simple carbs like sugar and alcohol.

How It Works Fat is more than twice as dense as protein and carbs. Thus dieters can consume the same amount of food but still lose weight if they eat less fat. Lots of complex carbs like whole grains help stabilize blood sugar, and lots of fiber increases satiety.

Downside Giving up meat is hard enough, but no fatty nuts or avocados?

When Lite Gets Heavy Low-fat foods can pack a high-fat wallop. Let the buyer beware!

It would be easier to count calories if we could just see the pesky things—you'd never have to eat a single one more than you want to. But calories are very good at hiding themselves—never more so than at health-food restaurants. Almost everyone has had the experience of bypassing a McDonald's for a virtuous, diet-friendly place, only to leave feeling more stuffed than if you'd just had the Big Mac and fries. That's no illusion. Menus at restaurants that claim to offer healthy alternatives are often booby-trapped with hidden fat and calories.

The bad *Nachos and cheese are high in fats*

Take those heart-healthy symbols you see next to menu offerings. A 2003 study in the *Journal of Marketing* found that diners may trust the little icons more than their own common sense, believing that there's a reduced risk for heart disease even if the symbol is next to a manifestly fatty food like lasagna. We're also suckers for the term low cholesterol, thinking that it's synonymous with low fat, which is by no means always the case.

Even when we make the right choice, we can trip up. If we're having a healthy entrée, we decide we might as well pile on the extras, loading up a salad with cheese or too much dressing. Healthy snacks can also mislead us. One study showed that if you give people the low-fat, low-calorie version of a food like a granola bar or Chex Mix, they'll take advantage of the benefit by eating 28% more of it than they would of the higher-fat version.

Perhaps worst of all, there's the notorious what-the-hell effect. Calorie counters who realize they're exceeding their limit often don't pull back to contain the

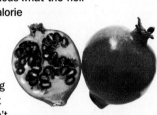

The good *Pomegranates are high in antioxidants*

damage but reason that the day is a dietary loss, so they might as well have fun, loading up on desserts and sides they'd otherwise avoid.

What can we do? First, keep alternative options in mind. A 2005 study showed that people are actually more likely to choose a lower-fat cheesecake when it appears on a menu alongside a high-fat version, almost as if picturing that dense serving of after-dinner indulgence makes the lighter choice more appealing. Having a real sense of serving size and calorie content can help too. Most studies suggest that only 10% to 20% of people know how to count calories. When the rest of us bother to guess, we usually lowball what's in a meal by as much as 45%.

One good idea: order what you want but push your plate away while you've still got a sizable portion left.

Finally, don't be too pure. There's nothing that

The ugly *But we love 'em too! Enjoy—infrequently*

makes food harder to resist than being told you can never have it. The occasional, moderate-size serving of warm chocolate cake or McDonald's fries is not going to kill you. And in case you forgot, it will be utterly delicious.

41

Command and Control

Bodywide web: the brain, nervous system and senses

ONGRATULATIONS: YOU NOW HAVE ONE MILLION more neurons than you did a second ago. And a second from now, you'll have one million more. Of course, your neurons are dying off at the same time. These neurons, along with the synapses that connect them, are the workhorses of the brain, tiny electro-chemical transmitters that keep the body running, receive information passed along from our sense organs and send out instructions to our muscles and other organs via the nervous system.

Altogether, these neurons account for only about 2% of your adult body weight, yet they consume up to 25% of the energy you produce each day. If that seems like an unreasonable share, consider that the figure was closer to 60% during the first year of your life. And though your brain stops growing in size by age 20, it never stops forming new circuits for as long as you live.

This three-pound lump of wrinkled tissue is about the size and shape of a cauliflower, and it's 85% water. The invaluable organ serves not only as the motherboard for every other system in the body, it is also the seat of your mind, your thoughts, your sense that you exist at all. You have a liver. You have your limbs. But you *are* your brain. It is the source of emotions, the repository of memory, the connection to our senses, the director of our appetites and pleasures. Yet this Great Oz of our existence remains, even now, shrouded behind curtains of mysterious molecules and mechanisms that continue to both bewilder and fascinate us.

As 21st century science exposes the workings of the brain to us as never before, imaging technologies are turning accepted truths on their head. We're finding that early brain scientists were at least partly right to think of the brain as a bordered organ, subdivided into zones and functions. But the lines are blurrier than they,

The brain is the seat of your mind, your thoughts, your sense that you exist at all. You have a liver. You have your limbs. But you *are* your brain

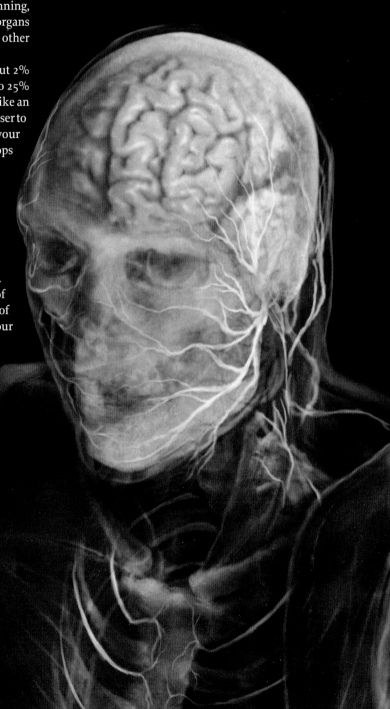

or we, ever imagined. Lose your vision, for example, and the tightly networked neurons that processed light may repurpose themselves to enhance other senses. Suffer a stroke in the area that controls your right arm, and Good Samaritan nerve cells from another region may take up at least some of the slack.

We're also learning about specialized neurons that allow us to mirror the behavior of people around us, which may be critical in helping us to learn such primal skills as walking and eating, as well as how to become social, ethical beings. The mystery of memory is being teased apart, exposing the way we store facts and experiences in addition to the emotional flavors associated with them. Magnetic resonance imaging is probing the brain as it operates, essentially—if still crudely—reading our minds, and raising all the ethical questions that attend such scientific clairvoyance.

Yet it would be a mistake to examine the brain in isolation, for its functions demand that it be intimately connected to the entire body. We call that essential sensory matrix the nervous system. The brain's partners in absorbing experience are the exquisitely tuned mechanisms of the sensory organs: the eyes, the nose, the senses of touch, smell and taste. Thanks to new technology, we can now map the areas of the brain where sensory information is processed. The bodywide web operates primarily through the brain and spinal cord and extends its grid of neurons everywhere, taking in information from sense organs, directing the operation of skeletal muscles, monitoring and regulating the body's internal organs and processes.

If you want to give your brain and nervous system a workout, while you explore their inner workings— have your brain direct your hands to turn the page. ■

Nerve grid *The brain and the spinal cord are the two primary organs of the nervous system*

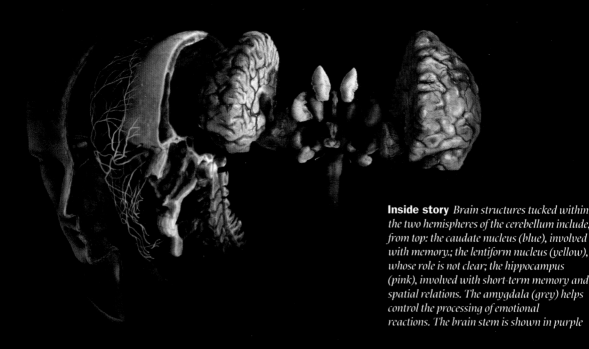

Inside story *Brain structures tucked within the two hemispheres of the cerebellum include, from top: the caudate nucleus (blue), involved with memory.; the lentiform nucleus (yellow), whose role is not clear; the hippocampus (pink), involved with short-term memory and spatial relations. The amygdala (grey) helps control the processing of emotional reactions. The brain stem is shown in purple*

Swaddled within three protective membranes in the skull, the brain is the most complex organ of the body. Driving its constant activity are the infinitesimal electrochemical transmitters called neurons. Throughout your lifetime, these hard-working nerve cells are constantly being born and dying off, in an endless cycle of growth and pruning that defines our intellectual development. Four weeks after conception, the embryo's neurons are already forming at an astonishing rate: 250,000 each minute. By 8 months, a baby's brain holds 1,000 trillion synapses, the vital junctions that connect neurons. By age 10, those synapses drop down to about 500 trillion, under a "use it or lose it" principle that prunes away underutilized connections to make the most active ones stronger. The brain is thus sculpted by experience: researchers found that when mothers spoke to their infants often, their children learned almost 300 more words by age 2 than did children whose mothers rarely spoke to them.

The brain consists of three primary regions: the forebrain, midbrain and hindbrain. The cerebrum, part of the forebrain, forms the hub: this control room for our memory, imagination, communication and reason takes up some 80% of the organ's total mass. It is divided into two halves, or hemispheres, each with special functions. The left half controls speech,

language and calculation; the right is responsible for spatial abilities, facial recognition and more.

Each hemisphere is further divided into frontal, parietal, occipital and temporal lobes. The frontal lobes dictate conscious thought and control voluntary movement, while the parietal lobes receive incoming data from the body's sensory organs and manage abstract mental functions, such as reading and math. The occipital lobes are specialized visual centers, while the temporal lobes help manage sensory memories, especially those associated with sound.

Moving down the brain toward the spine, brain functions become more reflexive and less cerebral. The midbrain holds several small organs of the limbic system: the thalamus, hypothalamus, subthalamus and epithalamus control the autonomic nervous system, which regulates involuntary systems such as the beating of heart muscles, our blood pressure, body temperature and sleep patterns.

The hindbrain, or brain stem, is located between the spinal cord and the brain and ferries information between the two structures, helping monitor and regulate such unconscious processes as breathing and heart rate. The two lobes of the cerebellum (Latin for "little brain") fit directly under those of the cerebrum and control muscle movement and posture. ■

Common Brain Diseases and Disorders

Stroke A break in normal brain function that occurs when a region receives insufficient blood flow, either because an artery is blocked or breaks opens and bleeds into the brain, and is thus starved of oxygen and nutrients.

■ **Symptoms** *Sudden confusion or trouble with walking, speaking or understanding speech; difficulty seeing in one or both eyes; dizziness, loss of balance; sudden severe headache.*

■ **If symptoms occur** Seek emergency medical attention quickly. Many primary care centers now use "clot-busting" drugs to unlock the artery. Long-term treatments include drugs to thin the blood.

Brain Tumor Abnormal tissue growth inside the skull, which can be either benign (noncancerous) or malignant (cancerous). Even benign tumors, however, can exert harmful pressure on sensitive tissues and interfere with normal brain function.

■ **Symptoms** *Headaches, seizures, nausea and* vomiting; difficulty in seeing or hearing; cognitive, motor and balance problems.

■ **Treatment** Surgery, radiation therapy or chemotherapy, or a combination of these approaches.

Encephalitis and Meningitis
Inflammation of the brain (encephalitis) or its surrounding tissues and the spinal cord (meningitis), usually caused by infection.

■ **Symptoms** *For encephalitis: nausea and vomiting, confusion, disorientation, drowsiness, seizures, stupor or coma. For meningitis: sudden fever, severe headache, stiff neck.*

■ **If symptoms occur** Immediate, aggressive medical intervention is imperative. Both diseases can progress quickly and have the potential to cause severe, irreversible neurological damage.

Victim *In May 2008, Senator Edward Kennedy was found to have malignant glioma, a cancerous brain tumor*

The Brain Terms to Know

Amygdala Small structure in the midbrain; part of the limbic system, it regulates the fear reflex.

Brain stem Also called the hindbrain, it is the major route by which the forebrain transmits information to and from the spinal cord and peripheral nerves.

Cerebellum Twin-lobed portion of the hindbrain that helps regulate posture, balance and coordination.

Cerebral cortex The outer layer of the cerebral hemisphere, it processes our conscious actions, including perception, emotion, thought and planning.

Forebrain The largest division of the brain, it includes the cerebral cortex and basal ganglia. The forebrain is the area devoted to the higher intellectual functions.

Hippocampus A forebrain structure involved in emotions, motivation, learning and memory.

Limbic system A set of brain structures that generate feelings, emotions and motivations, it is essential to learning and memory.

Plasticity The ability of the brain to change its structure and function within certain limits, through the formation or strengthening of connections between neurons.

Positron emission tomography (PET) Technique for imaging regions of the brain while they are active.

Sources (2): National Institutes of Health

Eight Common Myths of the Brain

1. Most humans use only 10% of their total brainpower.

Fact Most humans use 100% of the brain's resources.

2. You learn things better when you are either asleep or deeply relaxed.

Fact Most evidence says we learn things most efficiently when we are alert and mentally focused.

3. The brain absorbs information like a sponge and reaches a natural limit when it is "saturated" with data.

Fact The brain's capacity to learn is almost limitless.

4. The brain is a blank slate, molded only by experience.

Fact Human infants are born with a library of reflexes and instincts, and genetics plays a significant role in how the brain develops.

5. The brain stops growing relatively early in life.

Fact True but misleading. The brain reaches its maximum weight and mass by age 20, but it continues to form new nerve connections until the last moments of life.

6. Brain cells, once damaged or destroyed, can never be replaced.

Fact Brain cells regenerate themselves constantly; researchers are hoping to identify new therapies to enhance this renewals process.

7. Human personality is largely determined by right-brain or left-brain dominance.

Fact Personality and other higher brain functions are shaped by both "sides" of the brain and reflect a host of additional influences.

8. Babies who listen to classical music and educational TV shows learn better.

Fact: Studies show exposing infants to stimulating videos and music have little impact on cognitive development, and in some cases, may even delay the learning of new words.

■On the Horizon Briefs

Migraine and Women
Women may be more sensitive to electrical brain charges

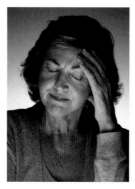

Three times as many women as men suffer from migraine headaches, a painful constriction and dilation of blood vessels in the brain often associated with the menstrual cycle, and UCLA researchers think they now know why. A 2007 study—while admittedly one conducted only on mice—showed that females have a lower tolerance to cortical-spreading depression (CSD), an electrophysiological wave that can propagate through the cortex of the brain. In men, CSD is less likely to lead to nausea, visual auras and pain, symptoms that women more commonly experience and that are the hallmarks of a migraine. The good news: in trials, drugs that block CSD waves show early success among female migraine victims.

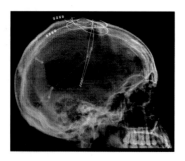

Rewiring the Brain A little bit of current can help awaken damaged minds

The X-ray image above shows a pair of electrodes implanted by doctors at the Cleveland Clinic into the brain of a 38-year-old man who had suffered severe brain damage in a 1999 mugging and had spent eight years in the dark cognitive well called a minimally conscious state. The electrodes were inserted into his thalamus, a deep, intact structure that could, in theory, jump-start the surviving circuits in the damaged cerebral cortex above it. When very low current was sent through the wires, it indeed awakened the man's higher brain: he can now identify objects and hold brief conversations.

The new treatment is called deep-brain stimulation (DBS), and it has already proved itself as a treatment for the tremors of Parkinson's disease. In 2008 DBS was under FDA consideration to treat obsessive-compulsive disorder and was in clinical trials to treat depression. Studies suggest it could also help control symptoms of Alzheimer's disease, epilepsy and some addictions. As of late 2007, some 40,000 people had undergone DBS treatment for Parkinson's; doctors stress it can help alleviate symptoms of the disease but not cure it.

Of Mice and Men A new atlas shows minds at work

You might think a mouse's brain would be of little help in explaining the workings of the human brain. The mouse brain is tiny—it weighs just 0.02 oz., compared with the 3-lb. human version—and a mouse's intelligence is just as feeble. Yet the genes responsible for building and operating both organs are 90% identical—so the mouse brain can be a powerful tool for unraveling the mystery of human mental disorders.

That's the idea behind the Allen Brain Atlas (ABA). Launched in September 2007 with $100 million from Microsoft co-founder Paul Allen, the atlas is the first Web-based, public-access database of all 20,000 or so genes expressed in the mouse brain. Want to see where in the brain specific genes are active? The ABA shows you, in vivid three-dimensional color (active genes are bright red in the image below). Curious about what types of brain cells are actively expressing a particular gene? The atlas provides molecular-level data that tell you. The site also contains an accounting of the genes in the mouse spinal cord, and a catalog of human brain genes has already begun.

As hits on the site multiply, researchers are using the atlas in their quest to develop new treatments for such human neurological disorders as dementia, schizophrenia and Alzheimer's disease. They've already identified a group of genes involved in age-related memory loss and have developed five compounds that mimic the activity of the genes. At least three of the new compounds appear to enhance memory function in aging rats.

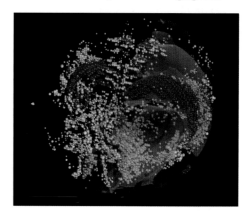

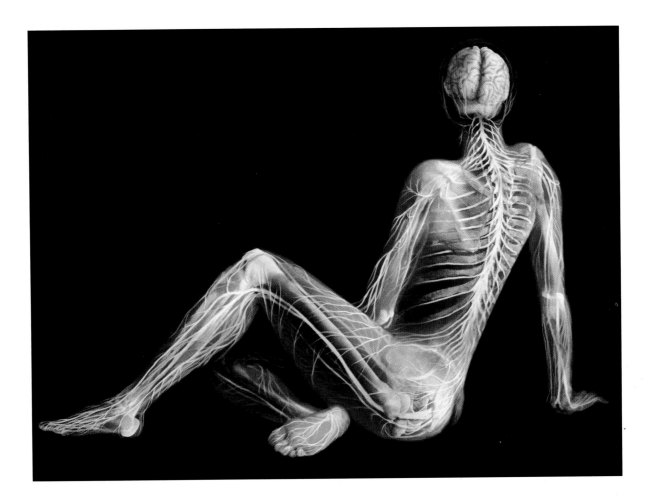

The Nervous System All wired up

SINCE THE DAWN OF THE INDUSTRIAL REVOLUTION, humans have compared their bodies to machines: muscles work like levers, the heart functions like a pump, and the lungs take on the work of an oxygen-generating bellows. The nervous system, however, is far more sophisticated, and its complex network of connections makes it less a workaday structure and more of a communications hub, an Internet of the body.

And what an information highway it is: more than 45 miles of wiring alone are devoted to connecting your brain to your skin. Many more miles link every other organ and system in your body to the 3-lb. central processing unit inside your skull. And it's electricity that carries the messages along the neurons and across the synapses that are the building blocks of the nervous system. These lines are always constantly thrumming with activity, relaying upwards of 3 million messages every second between your brain and every point in your body at speeds of up to 170 m.p.h.

Like any elegant network, the nervous system is built on radiating branches and forks. At its hub sits the central nervous system, which consists of the brain and the spinal cord. These two main organs of the nervous system are wired to every other part of the body. As information from the external world enters the body though our sensory organs—sounds from the ear, sights from the eye, tastes and smells from the tongue and nose, and so on—the nerves carry them to the brain.

The nervous system monitors our inner world as well, receiving input from every internal organ and system of the body and keeping the brain in constant touch with systems that are humming along well or those that are faltering to keep up. Finally, the nerves carry the messages that direct all our responses, from simple, unconscious reflexes like the act of blinking when a speck of dust lands in your eye to the enormously complicated set of nerve-muscle interactions that go into executing a perfect golf swing. ∎

Anatomy Lesson The Nervous System

The brain and spinal cord are the two primary nerve centers of the body, to which all nerve roads lead. Because of their primacy, they are regarded as a system unto themselves—the central nervous system. Where this central system ends, the peripheral nervous system begins. Encompassing all the other nerve tissue in your body, this grid starts with 12 pairs of cranial nerves that extend from the brain to the head and neck, where they control motor and sensory systems.

Below the skull, the peripheral system includes 31 pairs of spinal nerves, which extend outward from the spinal cord to the rest of the body. Because the spinal cord is the single most important nerve in your body, it is also the best protected: three layers of strong tissue, separated by shock-absorbing fluid and surrounded by the hard bones of the vertebrae, envelop it. Injuries or severance of the spinal cord can result in paralysis due to the inability to send nerve signals from the brain along the spinal cord to the muscles.

The 31 spinal nerves fall into four major categories: from top to bottom, cervical nerves connect to the shoulders, arms, hands and diaphragm; thoracic nerves to the chest and abdomen; lumbar nerves to the lower back and parts of the leg; and the sacral nerves to the buttocks, genitals and most areas of the legs and feet.

The peripheral nervous system is divided into the somatic and autonomic nervous systems. The somatic system controls voluntary muscle movements and sends sensory information from most parts of the body to the brain. The autonomic system oversees the involuntary functions of organs and glands.

The last important divisions are the two halves of the autonomic nervous system, the sympathetic and para-sympathetic systems. The first system switches on during moments of crisis or excitement and governs instinctive metabolic reactions, like the "fight or flight" response. The second is at work during ordinary moments, helping conserve energy and regulate the metabolism, which gives rise to its reputation as "the rest and digest" part of the nervous system.

Almost all tissue in the nervous system consists of two types of cells. Neurons perform the glamorous work of receiving incoming sensory information and transmitting nerve impulses to and from the brain and throughout the body. Less well known are the neuroglia cells, or glial cells, which serve as the glue that holds the nervous system together by providing neurons with nutrients, protection and other forms of support.

Contrary to widespread perception, not every movement in the body originates in the brain. Some, such as the patellar reflex (the "knee-jerk response," triggered in a doctor's office when a small hammer taps the middle of the leg), are hard-wired into the spinal cord itself. The impulses registering the hammer's impact travel only as far as the spinal cord, before the command to respond by contracting the tissue is sent back. The process is thus brainless, if not painless.

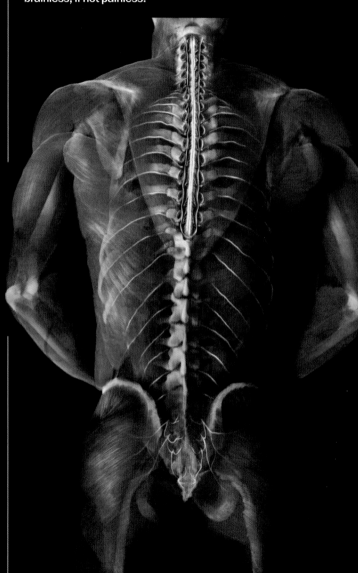

Pathways *The spinal cord, with the brain, makes up the central nervous system; above, it is exposed within the vertebrae. Spinal nerves branch out from the cord to the rest of the body*

Nerves Terms to Know

Axon A long, branching outgrowth of a neuron, it carries nerve impulses to other cells. Each neuron has a single axon.

Dendrite A branching outgrowth of a neuron, it carries nerve impulses into the cell body, the central hub of the neuron. Each nerve has many dendrites.

Glial cells Specialized cells that surround and support neurons.

Motor neuron A neuron that delivers information to muscles or glands.

Myelin The fatty sheath that surrounds and insulates axons.

Nerve A bundle of neurons bound together by a protective blanket of connective tissue.

Neural pathway An interconnected set of neurons, similar to a bus route, that delivers information for a specific body function, such as bending the knee or lifting a finger.

Neuron The basic cells of the nervous system that transmit sensory information throughout the body in the form of electric charges.

Neurotransmitter A chemical produced by neurons that carries messages to other neurons.

Sensory input Information received by the body through the sense organs: eyes, ears, nose, tongue and skin.

Stimulus Any information coming into the body that generates a nerve impulse.

Source (2): National Institutes of Health

Common Nerve Diseases and Disorders

Amyotrophic Lateral Sclerosis A rapidly progressing, fatal disease that attacks the nerve cells that control voluntary muscles.

■ **Symptoms** *Twitching or cramping in one area of the body (especially hands or feet), followed by loss of voluntary muscle control in that area, which later spreads to all other regions of the body.*

■ **Treatment** ALS is incurable and fatal, and there is no standard course of treatment. However, the FDA has approved the first drug treatment for the disease, riluzole, which is believed to reduce damage to motor neurons and prolong survival by several months.

Epilepsy A disorder in which groups of neurons fire abnormal signals.

■ **Symptoms** *Abnormal sensations, emotions and behavior, often including convulsions, muscle spasms, seizures and loss of consciousness.*

■ **Treatment** There is no cure, but in most cases, drugs and surgical techniques can control seizures.

Multiple Sclerosis A disease of the central nervous system that disrupts signals between the brain and other parts of the body.

■ **Symptoms** *Signs include vision problems, muscle weakness and impaired coordination; and numbness or "pins and needles"*

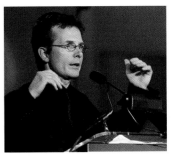

Advocate *Actor Michael J. Fox, a Parkinson's victim, has become a spokesman for those afflicted*

in extremities. Advanced MS can result in paralysis.

■ **Treatment** There is no cure, but medications such as steroids and immune modulators can help control symptoms.

Parkinson's Disease A progressive motor system disorder that that can cause minor tremors or severe disability.

■ **Symptoms** *Trembling in hands, arms, legs, jaw and face; stiffness of the limbs and trunk; slowness of movement; difficulty maintaining balance and coordination.*

■ **Treatment** There is no cure yet, but medications such as levodopa and carbidopa can provide relief from the symptoms. The FDA is also reviewing the benefits of a new therapy, deep brain stimulation (DBS), a procedure in which implanted electrodes send pulses to the brain to override faulty impulses.

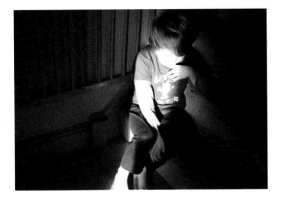

Autism: What Epidemic?

Is the U.S. in the throes of an epidemic of autism, a disorder that retards brain development in children? Statistics say yes: before 1990, autism was reported to affect just 4.7 out of every 10,000 American children, but by 2007, it was striking 60 per 10,000, according to many estimates—the equivalent of 1 in 166 kids. In his 2007 book, *Unstrange Minds: Remapping the World of Autism*, George Washington University anthropologist Roy Richard Grinker persuasively argued that much of this surge can be explained by social factors, including broader definitions of the disease, the reduction of the stigma around it and policies that offer financial rewards to parents of victims and their schools.

Briefing The Senses

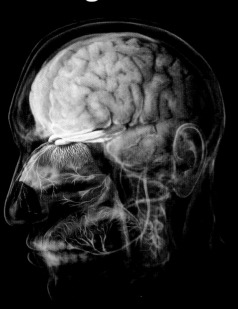

Taste and Smell

Throughout human evolution, the sense of smell was crucial to early human survival, and the abililty to sniff danger still warns us away from many hazards, be it smoke from a fire or spoiled food containing toxic bacteria. Smell and its partner, taste, are the senses that provide some of our most visceral interactions with the world.

Our sense of smell is roughly 10,000 times more sensitive than our ability to taste—which is why most of what we experience as taste is actually through the way things smell. The 10,000 or so taste buds on the tongue, the inside of the cheeks and the upper part of the throat register only five basic sensations: sweet, sour, bitter, salty and umami (a little-known taste triggered by certain acids). Yet the taste buds can distinguish between many thousands of separate odors.

The chemistry of smell takes place in a microscopic layer of mucus in the nose that covers tiny, hairlike nerves sprouting from the olfactory receptors. When tiny particles bearing odor enter the nose, they are intercepted and absorbed by this mucous covering, which contains highly specialized nerve cells. When a layer of mucus designed to recognize the smell of roses, for example, finds a particle that matches its profile, the nerve beneath the mucus sends a message to the brain. Just a few molecules—a mass amounting to a handful of atoms—can fire the appropriate receptor. And because smell is directly linked to the part of the brain that processes memory and emotion, a familiar aroma can trigger a decades-old flood of vivid feelings.

Hearing

Sounds are actually vibrations, and before we can hear anything, the vibrations have to be transformed into signals that specialized structures in the ear can pick up and relay to the brain. The process begins in the outer ear, where a flap of skin called the auricle, or pinna, funnels sound waves, amplifying and guiding them from the outer ear into the ear canal. Once inside, the vibrations take a three-stage journey. The first stage begins at the tympanic membrane, or eardrum, which vibrates in response to sound waves. These movements unleash a domino-like response by the ossicles, the trio of bones in the middle ear that are shaped like a hammer, anvil and stirrup. Each time one of them moves, it passes the vibration to the next bone in line.

Their activity, in turn, causes tremors in the oval window, a layer of tissue at the border of the inner ear. This curling, mazelike chamber of bone includes the snail-shaped, fluid-filled cochlea. The vibrations are then translated to waves within the fluid, stimulating the Organ of Corti, a spiral-shaped structure that contains thousands of microscopic hairs that move in response to the waves. Their agitation fires one or more of the 20,000 or so auditory receptor nerves within the Organ of Corti, creating a nerve impulse that shuttles to the brain and is interpreted as sound.

In addition to helping us hear, the inner ear keeps our body in balance, thanks to another set of fluid-filled structures, the semicircular canals. Like the Organ of Corti, these tubes contain microscopic hairs that react to the body's position and transmit this information to the internal gyroscope in the brain.

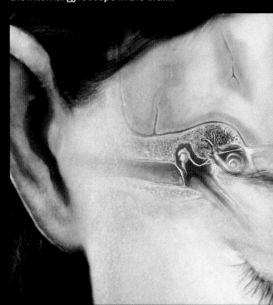

▨ Touch

No sensory system bombards the brain with more information than touch. Millions of nerve cells, arrayed over every inch of your body's surface and beneath it as well, constantly send impulses to the central nervous system. For this reason, no sense is more routinely ignored or selectively heeded: we aren't conscious of the pressure exerted by our clothing, but the instant our nerves detect significant pain in the body, multiple parts of the sensory system switch into high alert.

The sense of touch is based on the responses of four types of specialized nerve cells, or receptors, that respond to pressure, pain, heat and cold. Because pain is the sensation most directly related to safety and survival, more than 90% of all our touch receptors are attuned to pain. The firing of pain receptors triggers reflexes that respond to danger before the sensation even reaches the brain. The discomfort of a thorn pricking the skin on your finger travels only as far as the spinal cord before a message is sent back, causing you to pull the finger away. The same message eventually reaches the brain, which can allow or override the reflex, but in the intervening fraction of a second, the body has already been spared from further damage.

In some ways touch is the first sense: it becomes active in babies developing within the womb as early as eight weeks after conception. And it is the most richly active sense at birth: at a time when all evidence indicates that both hearing and vision are still a confusing blur, newborns respond in very precise ways to being touched. Studies show that babies who are not held, stroked and kissed often suffer from poor physical and mental health.

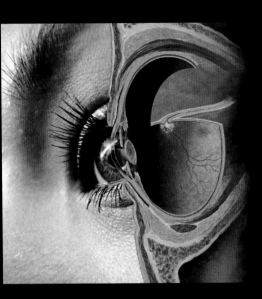

▨ Sight

The two small openings known as pupils, each centered in the middle of the eyeball, are your only windows on the world. As light shines or wanes, these pupils expand and shrink in response. In front of each pupil lies the lens, a disc-shaped transparent tissue that can be stretched and pulled into different forms by six straplike muscles, allowing it to focus light rays arriving from various distances on the back of the eyeball. That's where the retina lies, and where microscopic cells called photoreceptors translate light into nerve impulses.

Each eye contains some 130 million of these photo-receptors, which are divided into rods and cones after their shape. Rods distinguish shades of gray and detect shape and movement. Cones see colors, dividing up the spectrum into shades of green, red and blue.

Once it hits the retina, light is transformed into electrical impulses that travel along the optic nerves to the brain, where the rays are assembled into a coherent picture. This involves several corrections: because the focusing process of the lens flips the image it sees upside-down and "flops" it as well, reversing left and right, the brain flips and flops them back. And because our eyes are set a small distance apart, they send slightly different images to the brain, each of which lacks perspective. The brain melds the two images, synthesizing a single view in three dimensions from the original pair of 2-D images. It's the brain, too, that fills in many blank areas of images with what experience has trained it to expect. One reason that human beings are so good at finding animals and other familiar shapes in clouds is that the mind, as much as the eyes, is the author of our visions.

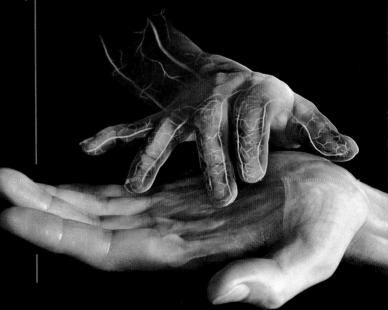

The Flavor of Memories

Scientists explore how emotions affect our recollections

LIKE ALMOST ALL MY CONTEMPORARIES, I STILL remember exactly where I was and what I was doing when John F. Kennedy was shot. It's so vivid, it's almost like watching a movie: I was home sick from fifth grade, lying on the couch in the living room. My mother had a talk-radio station playing. Suddenly a newscaster broke in with the news that shots had been fired in Dallas and that the President had been rushed to a hospital. Then a few minutes later came these precise words, spoken in just the tone you would imagine: "Ladies and gentlemen, the President is dead," followed immediately by funeral music. My mother burst into tears, and I, profoundly embarrassed, fled the room.

That scene, which I have replayed many times since 1963, perfectly illustrates two crucial facts that neurologists have come to understand in the past few years about the workings of human memory—facts that have important implications for the treatment of a variety of mental ailments, from posttraumatic stress to obsessive-compulsive disorder. The first is that, despite its movie-like clarity, my memory of J.F.K.'s assassination is almost certainly wrong in some details, and maybe even some significant ones. That's because I'm not simply calling up the original memory laid down in November 1963. I'm recalling the last time I thought about it. Each time we retrieve and re-store a memory, it can be subtly altered by all sorts of factors. What goes back into our brains is like the new version of a text document, overwriting the old.

The second fact: memory and emotion are intimately linked biochemically, with hormones like adrenaline actively involved in forming the neurological patterns we call memories. "Any kind of emotional experience will create a stronger memory than otherwise would be created," says James McGaugh, a neurobiologist at the University of California at Irvine. "We remember our embarrassments, our failures, our fender benders."

On the face of it, that doesn't seem so surprising: we feel strong emotion at important events, which are obviously more memorable than ordinary moments. But the connection is much deeper than that and dates back to our deepest evolutionary past. "The major purpose of memory," observes McGaugh, "is to predict the future." An animal that can remember the significance of that large, nasty-looking thing with the big teeth and sharp claws will survive longer and produce more offspring.

What happens biochemically, says McGaugh, is that when faced with an emotion-charged situation, such as a threat, our bodies release the stress hormones adrenaline and cortisol. Among other things, these signal the amygdala, a tiny, neuron-rich structure nestled inside the brain's medial temporal lobes, which responds by releasing another hormone, called norepinephrine. Norepinephrine does two important things. First, it kicks the body's autonomic nervous system into overdrive: the heart beats faster, respiration quickens, and the muscles tense in anticipation of a burst of physical exertion.

Second, even as it's kick-starting the body, the amygdala sends out a crackle of signals to the rest of the brain. Some of them put the senses on high alert, ready to deal with a threat. But these signals also tell the neurons that any memories recorded in the next few minutes need to be especially robust. One piece of evidence for this scenario: Lawrence Cahill, a colleague of McGaugh's at

> **'We remember our embarrassments, our failures, our fender benders.'**
> **—neurobiologist James McGaugh**

Irvine, showed subjects emotionally arousing film clips, simultaneously gauging the activity of their amygdalae using positron-emission tomography (PET) scans. Three weeks later, he gave the subjects a surprise memory quiz. The amount of amygdala activity predicted with great accuracy how well they remembered the film clips.

Imaging studies also make clear that it isn't just dangers or tragic events that cement memory formation. Positive emotions, also mediated through the amygdala, have the same effect. Again, that's a sensible evolutionary development. If eating or having sex makes you happy, you'll remember that and do it again, keeping yourself healthy and passing on your genes as well.

Virtually no expert doubts the connection between

Time changes *Article by* TIME *Science writer Michael Lemonick. At right, memories naturally grow hazier over time*

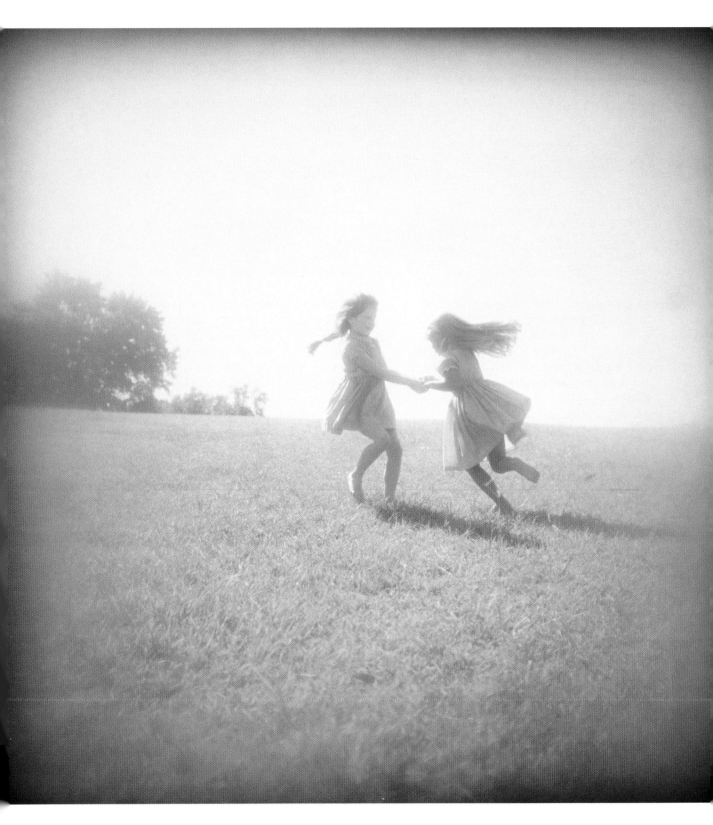

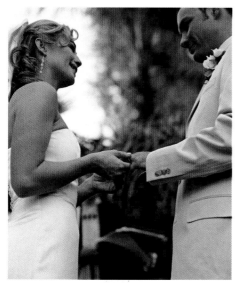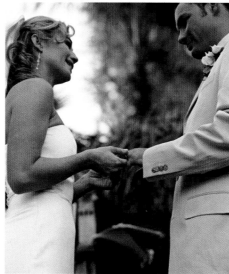

Memory lane *Happy events, like sad ones, burn themselves into our memories with the aid of neurotransmitters released by the amygdala in the brain. But over time, the details of memories can alter, for each time we access one, our brain is also booting up the last time we recalled it, like editing multiple versions of a computer text file*

the hormones of emotion and memory—and nobody doubts that memory can be enhanced artificially. It's not necessarily a good idea, though. Give someone a shot of adrenaline, and memory temporarily improves. But it also drives up the heart rate, so it could be dangerous for the elderly. Other memory enhancers, like Ritalin or amphetamines, used by college students to cram for exams, are highly addictive.

For people haunted consciously or unconsciously by painful memories, there may be hope. Roger Pitman, a professor of psychiatry at Harvard Medical School, is working to understand posttraumatic stress disorder (PTSD). The syndrome, he believes, is the result of brain chemicals reinforcing themselves in a cerebral vicious circle. "In the aftermath of a traumatic event," he says, "you tend to think more about it, and the more you think about it, the more likely you are to release further stress hormones, and the more likely they are to act to make the memory of that event even stronger."

That's consistent with McGaugh's ideas, but there are only a few bits of hard evidence so far to support it. One comes from Israel: researchers found that among people who showed up at emergency rooms after traumatic events, those admitted with the fastest heartbeats had the highest risk of later developing PTSD. Another is the surprising fact that after an accident, there's a much higher rate of PTSD in those with paraplegia (paralysis of the lower body) than in those who suffer quadriplegia (paralysis of all four limbs). "It doesn't make any psychological sense," says Pitman. But it makes physiological sense because quadriplegia severs the link between the brain and the adrenal glands.

To test his theory, Pitman went to the emergency room at Massachusetts General Hospital in Boston and intercepted patients who had suffered serious traumas. He gave some of them propranolol, a drug that interferes with adrenaline uptake. The rest got placebos. He also had them tape-record accounts of the traumas. When Pitman played back the tapes eight months later, eight of 14 placebo patients developed higher heart rates, sweaty palms and other signs of PTSD. None of the patients on the real drug had such responses.

Other compounds may work in similar ways. Michael Davis, a professor of psychiatry at Emory University in Atlanta, is about to launch a study of at least 120 soldiers returning from Iraq to see whether a compound called D-cycloserine could help prevent PTSD. This compound activates a protein that helps the mind form new, less emotional associations with the original trauma, letting patients tolerate the memory better. The theory behind D-cycloserine's function is consistent with cognitive behavioral therapy (CBT), currently the most effective non-drug technique dealing with phobias, PTSD and obsessive-compulsive disorder. CBT involves encouraging the patient to examine upsetting ideas and consciously assign new, more positive associations to them. Drugs like D-cycloserine may simply streamline the process.

Can we find a key to unlock the doors that open on the past? In recent years neurologists and psychopharmacologists have come up with dozens of medications to treat schizophrenia, depression and other disorders. The next batch of psychoactive drugs, such as those to control PTSD, could help heal the even more mysterious disorders of memory. ∎

■ **Briefing** Six Lessons for Understanding Stress

Take a deep breath. Now exhale slowly. You may not have noticed it, but your heart has just slowed down a bit; it will speed up again when you inhale. This regular-irregular beat is a sign of a healthy interaction between heart and head. Each time you exhale, your brain sends a signal down the vagus nerve to slow the cardiac muscle. With each new inhalation, the signal gets weaker and your heart revs up. Inhale, beat faster. Exhale, beat slower. It's an ancient rhythm that helps your heart last a lifetime. And it leads to lesson No. 1 in how to manage stress and avoid burnout.

No. 1 Remember to Breathe
Americans tend to cope with stress in all the wrong ways. We frequently deal with chronic stress by watching television, skipping exercise and forgoing healthy foods. But these coping mechanisms keep you from doing things that help buffer your stress load—like exercising or relaxing with friends or family—and may add greater stress to your body. Worse, using many of our most cherished time-saving gadgets can backfire. Cell phones and mobile e-mail devices, for example, make it harder to get away from the office to decompress.

No. 2 Stress Alters Your Body Chemistry
For years psychologists concentrated on the behavioral symptoms of burnout: lost energy, lost enthusiasm and lost confidence. Now, thanks to new brain scans and more sophisticated blood tests, scientists can directly measure some of the effects of stress on mind and body as adrenaline, cortisol and other neurotransmitters hit the bloodstream. Researchers are finding that the body's response to stress involves several interrelated pathways, and that posttraumatic stress disorder (PTSD), burnout, chronic fatigue syndrome and fibromyalgia are all related in physiological ways.

No. 3 You Can't Avoid Stress
Each morning the level of the stress hormone cortisol in our body rises as we await the new day. It peaks, then falls off—but not in those who suffer from severe depression, whose cortisol level remains high. Yet in the case of acute burnout victims, the cortisol response is blunted—a symptom also common among Holocaust survivors, rape victims and soldiers suffering from PTSD.

No. 4 Stress Can Age You Before Your Time
Scientists have long suspected that unremitting stress does damage to the immune system, but they weren't sure how. Recent tests of the white blood cells of mothers who had cared for children with disabilities, however, showed accelerated aging. The changes took place in microscopic structures called telomeres, which keep chromosomes from shredding.

No. 5 Stress Has No Favorites
Researchers have now found that subjects with low self-esteem are more vulnerable to stress, perhaps because the hippocampus organ in their midbrain, associated with memory, is small, contributing to cortisol buildup.

No. 6 There Are Many Ways to Relieve Stress
When we are under stress, when too many of the rules change or what used to work doesn't anymore, our ability to reason takes a hit. Yet simply being aware of our nervous system's built-in bias toward feeling helpless in the face of unrelieved stress can help us identify and develop healthy habits—like those in the box below— that will lighten at least some of the load.

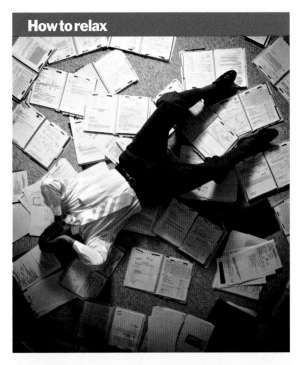

How to relax

Breathe deeply To relax the heart and reduce blood pressure

Take a vacation To clear your head and recharge your batteries

Make friends Social isolation amps up stress's psychological damage

Exercise regularly It protects the heart, which is often the first to feel the effects of stress

Eat healthy Fruits and veggies counter the inflammatory proteins created by stress

Rest easy Irregular sleep magnifies the effects of stress

Do what you love And if you can't love your job— find a hobby!

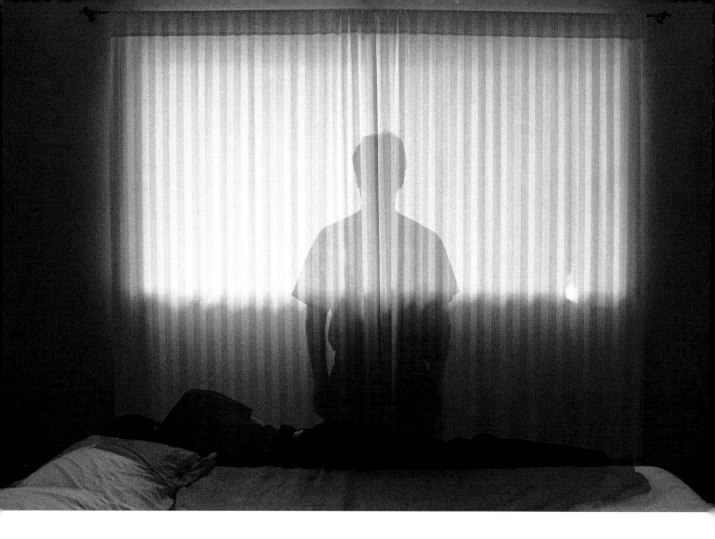

At the Hour of Our Death

Are near death experiences related to a form of sleep disorder?

THE STORIES ARE FAMILIAR BY NOW, YET NO LESS BIZarre for those who experience them. Patients lie at the point of death or very near it. Suddenly, their eyes are blinded by a powerful white light, even as they feel their spirit leaving their body and hovering above to observe it. Perhaps a tunnel is seen, beckoning them into the afterlife, or deceased relatives and divine figures appear. Patients may be guided by one of these spirits through a life review in which, some report, they feel again every emotion the past events aroused. Though they believe themselves to be dead, this cascade of feelings typically occurs against a prevailing sense of euphoria. At some point, they're told it's not their time and their spirit returns to the confinement of their body, most often through the top of the head.

Those who have lived through them say there is nothing hazy about these events, which we now call a near death experience (NDE). On the contrary, they are reported as seeming more real than real life, whatever that means. Most NDES change those who have them, dampening or obliterating any fear of death.

Such experiences have created a conflict in science, which centers not on whether they happen but on what they are. It's accepted, based on various studies, that between 4% and 18% of people who are resuscitated after cardiac arrest have an NDE. Researchers tend to fall into one of two camps on these events. The first argues that an NDE is a purely physiological event that occurs within an oxygen-starved brain. The second camp is as adamant that no theory based purely on the workings of the brain can account for all elements of an NDE, and that we should consider the mind-bending possibility that consciousness can exist independent of a functioning brain.

At present, more progress is being made by the scientists trying to solidify the brain-based theory of NDES. Their argument goes something like this: survival is our most powerful instinct. When the heart stops and oxygen is cut, the brain goes into all-out defense. Torrents of neurotransmitters are randomly generated, releasing countless fragmentary images and feelings from the temporal lobes that store memory. Perhaps the life review is the brain frantically scanning its memory banks for a way out of this crisis. The images of a bright light and tunnel could be due to impairment at the rear and the sides of the brain, respectively, while the euphoria may be a neurochemical antipanic mechanism triggered by extreme danger.

As for perhaps the strangest element of NDES, the out-of-body experience (OBE), studies led by Swiss neuroscientist Olaf Blanke have shed light on what may be occurring. In 2002, Blanke and others reported that they were able to induce OBES in an epilepsy patient by stimulating the brain's temporoparietal junction (TPJ), thought to play a role in self-perception. In instances where blood supply is cut, says Blanke, "the effects are occurring first at the TPJ, which is a classical watershed area of the brain." It's probable, he concludes, that stress in the TPJ causes the dissociation of NDES, one that in this view is entirely illusory.

What science has lacked until recently is an overarching theory that might explain why NDES seem so coherent. In two articles published in the science journal *Neurology*, a team of University of Kentucky researchers led by neurophysiologist Kevin Nelson proposed that NDES occur in a dreamlike state brought on when crisis in the brain trips a predisposition to a type of sleep disorder, REM intrusion. REM (rapid eye movement) sleep is the relatively active brain state in which most dreaming is thought to occur. REM intrusion is a disorder in which the sleeping person's mind wakes up before his body does. He feels awake, yet the muscle paralysis of REM can remain; he may also hallucinate until mind and body get back in synch. "Lay people think you're either awake or asleep," says Nelson, "but you needn't go directly from one to the other."

Some years ago, while studying firsthand accounts of NDES, Nelson read the story of a woman whom medical staff had written off as dead and whose attempts to protest she was alive were thwarted by paralysis. Paralysis? As also happens in REM intrusion? The seed of a new theory linking REM and NDES grew in Nelson's mind.

He tested it by comparing the frequency of REM intrusion in 55 people who'd had NDES with 55 who hadn't as controls. The results were striking: 60% of the first group reported some history of REM intrusion; 24% of the second. Nelson postulates that both REM intrusion and NDE involve a glitch in the arousal system that causes some people to experience blended states of consciousness. He stresses that he doesn't consider NDES to be dreams, rather that the NDEr "engages through the REM mechanism regions of the brain that are also engaged during dreaming," regions that infuse both dreams and NDES with emotion, memories and images.

Nelson's theory goes some way toward explaining how NDES can seem to occur when the brain is down. The sleep/wake switch is in the brainstem, which helps control the body's most basic functions and, when the patient is in cardiac arrest, stays active for longer than the higher brain. As for people reporting accurately on events that went on around them while they were apparently unconscious, Nelson says "they may be seemingly out of it but still processing in a very aberrant way."

Nelson's theory was picked apart by two veterans of the field who favor a more spiritual view of NDES. In a 2007 issue of the *Journal of Near-Death Studies*, oncologist Jeffrey Long and psychotherapist Janice Miner Holden argued that since 40% of NDErs in Nelson's study denied ever having had an episode of REM intrusion, the idea that it underlies NDES "seems questionable at best."

On balance, it's almost certain that NDES happen in the theater of one's mind, and that in the absence of resuscitation, it's the brain's final sound-and-light show, followed by oblivion. Nonetheless, there's still no definitive explanation. There mightn't be a ghost in the machine. But it's a machine whose complexities remain well beyond our grasp. ∎

The body's sleep/wake switch is in the brainstem, which in cardiac arrest stays active longer than the higher brain

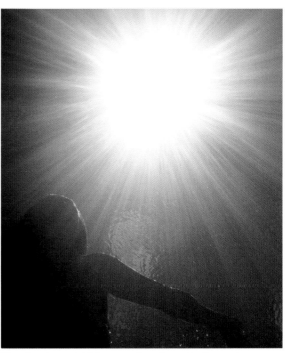

Illuminations *A high proportion of near death experiences includes the appearance of a blindingly white light, often at a tunnel's end*

■ On the Horizon Briefs

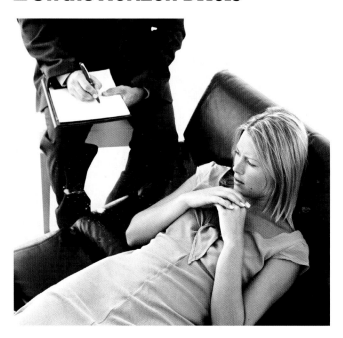

The Talking Cure In Australia, the couch makes a comeback for psychological woes

In the 1890s Sigmund Freud first postulated the family of psychological theories and methods that underpin the many forms of psychotherapy available today. It was Freud who first articulated the existence of the subconscious mind, which he said is shaped by early experience and can profoundly affect moods and behavior throughout life. Accessing this deep well, he said, is just a matter of remaining vigilant—patients would offer glimpses into the subconscious through dreams and slips of the tongue. But the arrival of new drugs for depression and psychosis in the early 1990s was a setback for psychotherapy, which some doctors began to portray as a chicken-soup remedy compared with the more sophisticated new magic bullets.

Now the pendulum may be swinging back. In Australia, the couch is gaining favor over pills as the main tool of treatment for many psychological ailments, with training institutions placing a stronger emphasis on psychotherapy. "We really want to get the balance right," said leading New Zealand psychotherapist Charles Le Feuvre, "and it may indeed be the case that things have gone too far away from psychotherapy." In recent years, proponents of psychoanalysis say, research has revealed the drugs' limitations and led to calls for a rethinking of the medication-based approach to treating depression. Aside from lifestyle changes, the only alternative for sufferers is some form of psychotherapy. "With drugs you can't even touch personality difficulties and maladjustment," Louise Newman, director of the New South Wales Institute of Psychiatry, said. Lately, she said, "we've reintroduced psychotherapy principles in the first year of training in order to returni to a more holistic approach" to treating mental distress.

Why meditate? It's good for what ails you, before it ails you

Researchers are continuing to discover how meditation can contribute to good health. At the hormonal level, studies have shown that meditation can counteract the fight-or-flight response that floods the body with the stress hormone cortisol and that also shuts down the parasympathetic system, which normally restores order after the alert is over. At a molecular level, meditation slows metabolism in red blood cells and suppresses the production of cytokines, proteins associated with the kind of heightened immune response often seen in stressed-out subjects.

And aside from slowing the heart rate, meditation may also reduce hardening of the arteries, especially in African Americans with high blood pressure. And there is growing evidence that a meditation program can have a positive, sustained effect on chronic pain and mood disorders, including depression and anxiety.

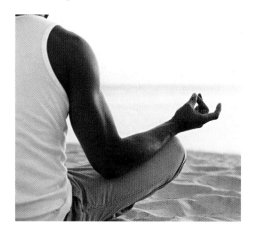

"While my training was in the science of the Western world, I also rely heavily on ... meditation to help my patients prepare for surgery," renowned cardiologist and author Mehmet Oz wrote in TIME. "Conventional medicine will keep breaking new ground in treatment and prevention, yet often the most effective solutions are found in the medicine cabinet of the mind. In one study, meditating 15 minutes twice daily reduced physician visits over a six-month period and saved the health-care system $200 a patient. Sometimes the best things in life *are* free."

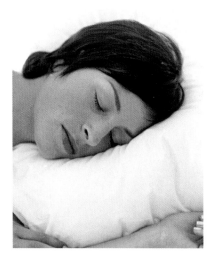

Slumber Gap Poor sleeping habits make women more susceptible to some diseases than men

Most women know that nothing kills a good complexion like a bad night's rest; there's a reason, after all, that it's called beauty sleep. If that's not motivation enough to keep up with your nightly shut-eye, here's another: doctors are learning that poor sleep habits may make women more vulnerable than men to heart disease and diabetes. A study by Dr. Edward Suarez at Duke University showed a consistent association between poor sleep and higher levels of the risk factors for heart disease and diabetes—but only among women. Men who had trouble falling asleep or had interrupted sleep did not show higher levels of the risk factors for developing the illnesses.

The results, published in the journal *Brain, Behavior and Immunity* in 2008, are among the first to link poor sleep to such a wide array of physiological changes. The study stopped short of establishing that a woman can reduce her risk for these conditions just by changing her sleep pattern, but it should galvanize women to pay more attention to the time they spend in bed.

The Listening Cure People who hear voices are finding new ways to cope

At age 7, Briton Peter Bullimore experienced his first auditory hallucination: a comforting voice that told him everything would be all right. By the time he was 10, he recalls, it had turned into 20 "threatening and demonic" voices; over the next two decades, they compelled him to steal, convinced him he was Jesus and persuaded him to attempt suicide. Years of psychiatric treatment offered no relief, so he joined a support group for people similarly afflicted. A decade later, he says, he is no longer at the mercy of his voices: "Now, when we argue, it's on my terms and not theirs."

Bullimore's recovery began with the Hearing Voices Network (HVN), an organization that brings such people together to exchange personal stories and coping strategies. Drawing on research by Dutch psychiatrists indicating that up to 1 in 25 people hears voices, as well as on studies suggesting that such auditory hallucinations emerge following traumas ranging from a parent's death to outright abuse, HVN seeks to recast the phenomenon as a normal experience. The group advises members to maintain a dialogue with their voices so they can live peacefully with and even appreciate their presence.

The HVN prescription flies in the face of traditional psychiatry, which prefers that patients take antipsychotic medication and ignore their voices, and warns that acknowledging them intensifies hallucinations. Dr. Cosmo

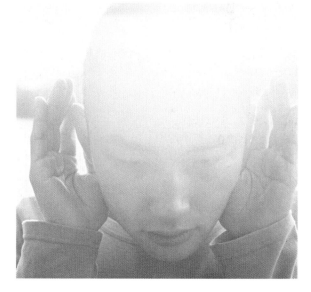

Hallstrom, a fellow at the Royal College of Psychiatrists in London, says hallucinations are usually symptoms of illness, particularly schizophrenia. He says that people who need psychiatric treatment don't always know it, and he worries that support groups like HVN could impede efforts to "combat the scourge of mental illness."

In about a third of cases, antipsychotic medication helps reduce distress, but for many it fails, says Dr. Sara Tai, a researcher at the University of Manchester in the U.K. The drugs also leave many patients feeling exhausted and emotionally numb, she maintains. For now, HVN offers an unusual approach that may benefit some.

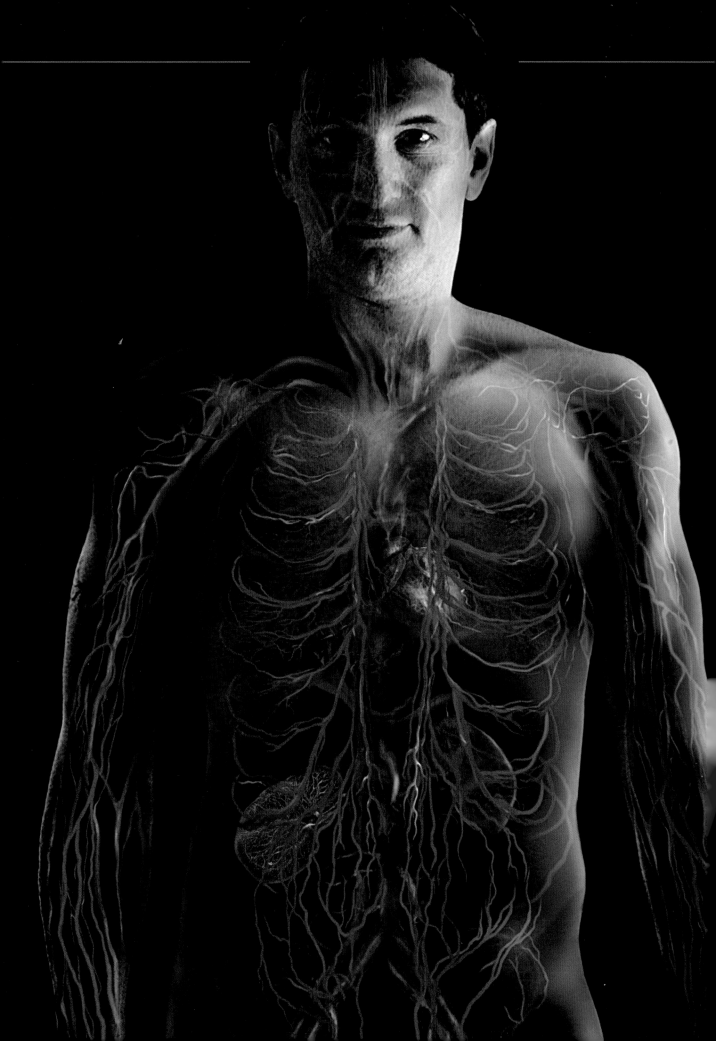

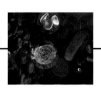

Dynamic Fluids

Highways through the interior: the circulatory system

WHEN FRENCH PHILOSOPHER BLAISE PASCAL DE-clared, "The heart has reasons of which reason knows nothing," he might have been describing an anatomical miracle that continues to mystify scientists. More than eight months before you were born, when your body was still no bigger than a grain of rice, a microscopic cluster of cells beneath your developing brain separated from the surrounding tissue and developed a unique ability to respond to electrical stimulus by contracting. These cells then arranged themselves into a flat sheet and began pulsing rhythmically.

A few weeks later, this flat sheet of cells folded over itself and formed a tube. A week after that, the tube sprouted a bulge in its midsection, which separated in a few days into two chambers. Months later, this chambered tube was beating 150 times each minute—a tiny fetal engine revved up to beat twice as fast as its mother's heart. Exactly which chemical instructions trigger this complex development remains a mystery, but that tube was the genesis of not only your heart but also your entire circulatory system.

In the following weeks, that clump of tissue grows into a muscle the shape of an upside-down pear and the size of your two clenched fists pushed together. Flexing more than 10,000 times each day, this powerhouse pushes the equivalent of more than 4,000 gal. of blood through your circulatory system every 24 hours. (That's enough to fill a bathtub more than 80 times over.) With each beat, your heart generates about two watts of electricity, and in a single hour, it produces and uses enough energy to lift a one-ton weight 3 ft. off the ground.

As the locomotive of the circulatory system, the heart is charged with moving blood cells first to the lungs, where they take on their load of oxygen, then along the more than 50,000 miles of vessels that stretch to every cell in the body—and then back for the return trip, depleted, for a recharge. The result of this brilliant design: the gallon and a half or so of blood in your body does a complete circuit out from your heart and back roughly three times each minute, traveling some 12,000 miles each day. Over your lifetime, your pounding, reliable heart will pump out some 1 million barrels of blood—enough to fill, well, a very long train of tank cars.

The network of vessels that conveys blood through your body is every bit as sophisticated as the pump that powers it. Arteries, which carry blood away from the heart, are sturdy conduits with thick, elastic, muscular tissue that take the force of surging blood pumped out at very high pressure. Veins, which carry blood back toward the heart under much lower pressure, have thinner walls and are equipped with a series of valves that keep the river of life moving in the right direction. These major vessels branch into capillaries, whose vanishingly thin walls allow them to pass oxygen and nutrients to individual cells in exchange for carbon dioxide and waste matter. The smallest capillaries are so slender that dozens could fit within the width of a human hair and so narrow that the blood flow within them slows down (for microscopically brief stretches of time) to a pace equivalent to one mile every 50 days, before speeding up once again on the way back to the heart. ∎

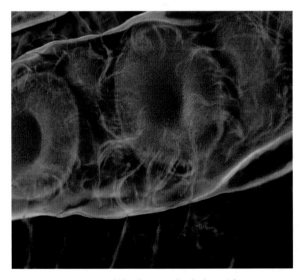

Special delivery *Red blood corpuscles, laden with oxygen, travel through the violet-hued capillary. Left: the major arteries and veins of the circulatory system connect the heart, lungs and kidneys*

Anatomy Lesson The Heart

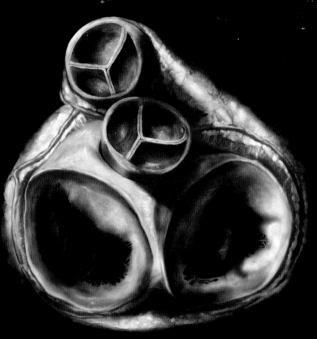

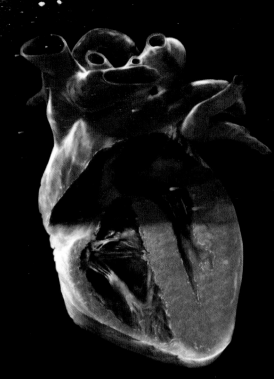

It's the ultimate in repetitive reliability. More than 100,000 times each day, more than 35 million times a year and more than a billion-plus times over a lifetime, your heart contracts, squeezing and pressuring the blood in your circulatory system another few inches along the more than 50,000 miles of arteries, veins and capillaries that stretch to every cell in your body. Constantly at work, even when you are at rest, the heart muscle exerts about twice as much force as your legs do when running—and keeps up this pace 24/7, every week of your life.

What makes this extraordinary feat possible? The muscle tissue of the heart is unlike any other in the body. Composed of long, stringy fibers, it does not require instructions from the brain to contract, although signals from the nervous system routinely cause the heart to pump faster or slower. Instead, its beating is triggered by its own miniature "brain," the sinoatrial node, which sends out regular electrical pulses to set off each heart contraction.

The heart is often called a stunningly efficient piece of natural machinery. True, but it is, in fact, *two* powerful natural machines. The right side of your heart pushes blood only as far the lungs, where it collects oxygen, then cycles it back into the left side of the heart. This second pump blasts this oxygen-rich blood out to the rest of your body through its network of arteries and capillaries. The

Four-part harmony *The heart is divided into four chambers: smaller atria on top, larger ventricles on the bottom. At left, four valves regulate blood flow into each of them. Blood enters the heart through the right atrium and flows into the ventricle, then is pumped to the lungs. The blood returns through the left atrium and is pumped to the rest of the body by the left ventricle. At right, a cross-sectional view shows that the left ventricle is the largest and most powerfully muscular of the four chambers*

returned blood carried by the veins is laden with carbon dioxide (CO_2) and other gaseous waste, which are expelled by the lungs, while solid cellular waste is filtered and expelled by the kidneys.

In addition to keeping us supplied with oxygen, blood passes through the intestines to pick up nutrients from food and deliver them to cells. The circulatory system also plays a vital role in the body's immune response, helps regulate vital functions like body temperature and maintains the pH balance in all our tissues.

Most of us instinctively reach for the left side of the chest to feel our hearts beat, but the heart lies almost directly in the center of the rib cage, tipped slightly forward and to the left, so the point at which the heart audibly taps against the chest wall is slightly off-center. Another misconception: the muffled two-step we call a "heartbeat" is not the sound of its muscles contracting but rather of its four valves opening and closing between contractions.

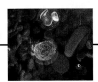

Common Circulatory Diseases and Disorders

Anemia A reduction in the number of oxygen-carrying red blood cells; or low levels of hemoglobin, the protein that carries oxygen from the lungs to all other parts of the body.

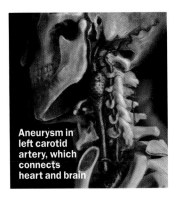

Aneurysm in left carotid artery, which connects heart and brain

■ **Symptoms** *Few early symptoms; later signs include fatigue, dizziness, headache; numbness in extremities; pale skin; rapid or irregular heartbeat, shortness of breath; chest pain.*

■ **Treatment** Changing diet, dietary supplements, blood transfusions.

Angina Chest pain or discomfort experienced when the heart muscle does not receive enough blood due to coronary artery disease (CAD), the most common form of heart disease.

■ **Symptoms** *Often felt as pressure or a squeezing pain in the chest but may also feel like indigestion or discomfort in the shoulders, arms, neck or back.*

■ **Treatment** Options range from drugs such as nitroglycerin to surgical interventions such as angioplasty.

Aneurysm An abnormal bulge in the wall of an artery, especially the aorta, which carries blood from the heart to the rest of the body.

■ **Symptoms** *Often undetected until the aneurysm bursts or blocks blood flow.*

■ **Treatment** "Watchful waiting" in mild cases; drugs to reduce swelling and pressures; and surgery to prevent rupture and repair arteries.

Coronary Artery Disease Occurs when the arteries that supply blood to heart muscle lose their flexibility and narrow as plaque, a buildup of cholesterol and other material, grows within artery walls.

■ **Symptoms** *Angina; shortness of breath or dizziness; sweating; heartburn, nausea or vomiting.*

■ **Treatment** Surgical procedures, including angioplasty or the installation of stents, are common, as is coronary bypass surgery.

Heart Attack Myocardial infarction most often occurs when a clot in the coronary artery blocks the supply of blood and oxygen to the heart, causing an irregular heartbeat, or arrhythmia, and a severe decrease in the heart's pumping power. More than 1 million Americans suffer heart attacks each year; approximately half of them die.

■ **Symptoms** *Pressure or pain in chest and upper body; nausea; dizziness.*

■ **If symptoms occur** Seek emergency care immediately. Many victims survive if treated within a few hours.

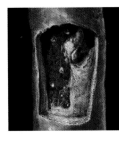

Plaque buildup in arteries (yellow)

Heart Failure The blanket name for any weakening of the heart's ability to pump enough blood, which is usually caused by CAD, high blood pressure and diabetes.

■ **Symptoms** *Blood and fluid backing up into the lungs; edema (buildup of fluid in the feet, ankles and legs); frequent fatigue; shortness of breath.*

■ **Treatment** Drugs or surgery; heart transplantation in extreme cases.

High Blood Pressure When blood exerts excess force against vessels.

■ **Symptoms** *The "silent killer" often exhibits no outward symptoms.*

■ **Treatment** Lifestyle changes to reduce stress, control weight, improve diet and fitness and cease smoking. Drug treatments include diuretics, beta blockers and vasodilators, which open the blood vessels.

Source: American Heart Association

The Heart
Terms to Know

Angiography X-ray test used to detect diseases of blood vessels.

Angioplasty Procedure to reopen blocked blood vessels to the heart. A catheter carrying a small deflated balloon is inserted in the affected artery. The balloon is threaded into the blockage, then inflated to widen the artery.

Arrhythmia Abnormal heartbeat caused by misfiring of electrical impulses.

Atrial fibrillation Rapid, uneven contractions in the heart chambers.

Beta blockers Drugs that reduce the heart's tendency to beat faster by blocking specific receptors on heart cells.

Congestive heart failure Weak pumping causes fluid retention and congestion in lungs.

Coronary artery bypass Surgical procedure to reroute blood around a blocked heart artery through a vessel grafted from elsewhere in the body.

Source: American Heart Association

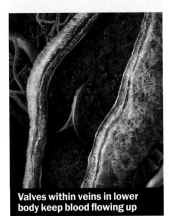

Valves within veins in lower body keep blood flowing up

THEVISUALMD.COM (5)

63

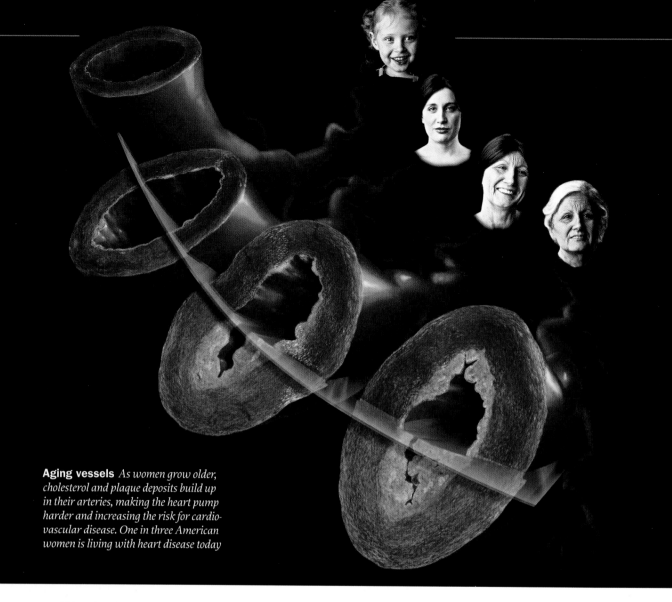

Aging vessels *As women grow older, cholesterol and plaque deposits build up in their arteries, making the heart pump harder and increasing the risk for cardiovascular disease. One in three American women is living with heart disease today*

■ **Briefing** Women and the Heart

Medical myths die hard, and one of the longest-standing holds that heart disease is a problem mostly for men. That's not even close to being true: according to the American Heart Association (AHA), more women than men die from heart disease in the U.S., and 1 in 3 women is living with it today. Yet despite these striking statistics, most patients and even many physicians still fail to think of heart problems when a woman complains of its classic symptoms: chest pain along with arm or jaw numbness. So in an attempt to reverse this faulty thinking and drive down mortality rates, in 2007 the AHA published a new set of guidelines for reducing women's risk of heart disease, heart attack and stroke.

One way to do it is with low-dose aspirin, already a well-known preventive for men. Women of any age who are at high risk for heart disease, says the AHA, should definitely consult their doctors about taking the blood-thinning painkiller daily. Women over 65 should do so

regardless of their health history—a reversal of the AHA's earlier guidelines. It gets trickier, though, for the average healthy woman under 65. In that population, aspirin doesn't help prevent heart attacks, although it can reduce the risk of nonbleeding types of stroke. (Men, by contrast, generally get little or no stroke-prevention benefit from aspirin.) The trick is for doctors to figure out on a case-by-case basis when the benefits of stroke reduction outweigh aspirin's risk of triggering bleeding in the stomach and the brain.

What's really noticeable about the new guidelines is the AHA's strong message about who's at risk—and that is almost every woman. Anyone who has at least one major cardiovascular-disease risk factor (including physical inactivity, poor diet and smoking) falls into that category. That leaves a scant 10% of U.S. women at what scientists call optimal risk, meaning they have no major risk factors.

"Our biggest message is, Don't wait until you have a

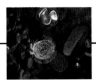

risk factor, because 40% of the time, the first symptom of heart disease for a woman is a fatal heart attack," warns Columbia University preventive cardiologist Dr. Lori Mosca, chair of the expert panel that wrote the updated guidelines.

In addition to new aspirin protocols, the guidelines add a recommendation to exercise 60 to 90 min., preferably daily, for women who are trying to either lose weight or sustain a weight loss. According to the U.S. Department of Health and Human Services, more than 60% of American women are overweight or obese—so again, most women need to comply with this new fitness prescription.

"We still have to answer the question of whether it's feasible to do an hour or 90 min. of exercise a day," admits Mosca, "but we also need to think about how to incorporate exercise into our everyday lives." Mosca, for instance, says she takes workout clothes to her son's sports events in case she can sneak in a few circuits around the track.

Alongside the list of dos, the guidelines also single out don'ts. Although it can have significant benefits for fetal development, folic acid, recommended just a few years ago, turns out not to help prevent heart disease and should not be used for that purpose. Neither should hormone-

'Our biggest message is, Don't wait until you have a risk factor. Forty percent of the time, the first symptom for heart disease in a woman is a fatal heart attack.'
—cardiologist Lori Mosca

replacement therapies or antioxidant supplements, such as beta-carotene and vitamins E and C. Omega-3 fatty-acid supplements, on the other hand, are a good thing, says the AHA.

If you're a woman and still not sure whether you should be concerned about heart-disease risks, whip out a tape measure and circle it around your waist. If it reads more than 35 in., chances are that you are at high risk for or already have high blood pressure, diabetes and/or high cholesterol. That means, it's time to talk to your doctor, make some lifestyle changes and get heart-healthy. That's one thing men and women also have in common: the basics still work. ■

Dos and Don'ts of a Healthy Heart

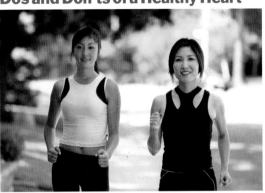

The American Heart Association suggests the following diet and exercise guidelines for reducing the risk of cardiovascular disease for the entire family.

Diet Guidelines
- Eat a variety of nutritious foods from all the food groups.
- Consume lots of vegetables and fruits. They are high in vitamins, minerals and fiber—and low in calories.
- Choose whole-grain, high-fiber foods. They contain fiber that can help lower your blood cholesterol and make you feel full, which may help you manage your appetite and weight.
- Minimize the intake of beverages and foods with added sugars.
- Reduce the saturated fat, trans fat and cholesterol content of your diet.
- Eat fish at least twice a week. Fatty fish like mackerel, lake trout, herring, sardines, albacore tuna and salmon are high in omega-3 fatty acids, which may help lower your risk of death from coronary artery disease.
- Choose lean meats and poultry without skin and prepare them without adding fats.
- Cut back on beverages and foods with added sugars, such as high-fructose corn syrup.
- Choose and cook foods with little or no salt.
- Eat less of nutrient-poor foods. Limit foods and beverages high in calories but low in nutrients. Read labels carefully—the Nutrition Facts panel will tell you how much of those nutrients each food or beverage contains.

Exercise Guidelines
Healthy adults aged 18 to 65 should engage in moderate-intensity aerobic physical activity for at least 30 min. on five days each week or vigorous-intensity aerobic physical activity for at least 20 min. on three days a week.

In addition, every adult should engage in activities that maintain or increase muscular strength and endurance, such as working with weights, a minimum of two days each week.

■ On the Horizon Briefs

Healing Hands No need to "talk to the hand." Now it talks to you

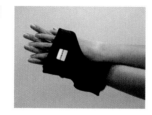

Cardiopulmonary resuscitation (CPR) always looks so dramatic on TV hospital shows: a shout of "Clear!" followed by a strategic thump to the chest—and another dead man is soon walking. But in reality, chest compressions are difficult to get right, even for trained health professionals. Enter the CPR Glove, a senior-year design project of three undergraduate engineering students from McMaster University. Once you slip it on, the black neoprene glove, which is embedded with sensors and chips, talks its wearer through the proper way to resuscitate by measuring the amount of pressure you exert with each compression as well as the frequency of your chest pumps. If you aren't pumping hard or fast enough, the glove instructs you to "compress faster." Not yet approved for use, the hands-on device is undergoing testing to measure its effectiveness.

From the Tummy to the Ticker A best-selling cardiologist has a prescription for you

After getting many Americans to embrace his South Beach Diet, cardiologist Arthur Agatston turned to territory closer to his medical practice in the 2007 best seller *The South Beach Heart Program* (Rodale). In an interview with TIME Health columnist Sanjay Gupta, M.D., Agatston argues we have become a nation too focused on treating heart disease and stroke rather than preventing them. Why? Because there isn't as much money to be made in prevention as there is in treatment.

Agatston's advice: take advantage of computed tomographic angiography (CAT), the noninvasive heart scan that takes about 10

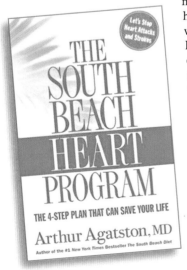

minutes and can tell you if you have any developing plaque in the vessels that supply blood to your heart. And invest in a sophisticated C-reactive protein test to measure the level of inflammation in your body. Cutting it down greatly reduces your chance of having a stroke or heart attack. Post-menopausal women over 50 should be sure to get these tests, as heart disease is the biggest killer of women. Agatston's last tip: work off any excess belly fat, an important predictor of heart disease. In short, get back to the basics: a healthy diet and frequent exercise.

Flipping Out? New research links stress to heart disease

The human heart does not like surprises. In the month after 9/11, incidents of dangerous heart rhythms in cardiac patients around New York City more than doubled. After a major 1999 earthquake in Taiwan, hospitalization for heart attacks skyrocketed near the epicenter. A private event such as the sudden death of a spouse can bring on grief so severe that sometimes our hearts, quite literally, break.

Researchers have long suspected that stress harms the body. But in part because individual reactions to stress are so variable, solid clinical evidence linking emotions to actual heart attacks and other coronary disease has been elusive. But that's changing. New studies suggest that both chronic strain at work and bad relationships put people at a markedly increased risk of heart trouble.

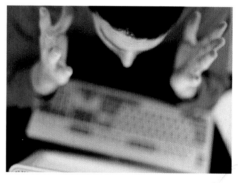

In a 2007 article in the *Journal of the American Medical Association,* researchers in Quebec reported that first-time heart-attack patients who returned to chronically stressful jobs were twice as likely to have a second attack as patients who found their work to be relatively stress-free. In another study published in 2007 in the *Archives of Internal Medicine,* University of London researchers said that British civil servants with stormy intimate relationships had a 34% higher risk of heart disease than those with more placid personal lives. The emotions at play in tense marriages can do cumulative damage to organs and tissues that may leave people at greater risk of illness, they wrote. As a result, researchers are calling for doctors to include the diagnosis and treatment of stress in routine care for patients with heart conditions.

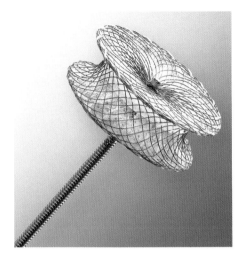

How Do You Mend a Broken Heart? A new patch helps stitch up ruptured cardiac muscles

Among the many dangers of a heart attack is damage to the walls of the heart. When cardiac muscle is stressed, ruptures between the usually separate left and right ventricles can cause blood to slosh back and forth between the two chambers, lowering its oxygen content. Surgery to repair the damage to the ventricles can be dangerous since, by definition, it's performed on a heart that is already weakened.

But doctors and patients now have a safer alternative, thanks to a new technique in which a polyester-coated metal patch is collapsed, threaded via catheter into the body and positioned in the heart to seal off the tear. This can buy patients the time they need to recuperate and allow them to postpone more extensive repair surgery. In many cases, it may even help them avoid that operation altogether, since the polyester covering on the patch encourages new heart tissue to grow, helping to permanently heal the rupture.

Where Party Meets Hearty College kids who binge drink may be doing long-term damage to their hearts

Binge drinking has always been a rite of college, but now it seems that kegger parties may have much more serious consequences than a hangover. Drinking heavily, it turns out—even for those as young as college students—could increase the risks of heart disease.

Research from the American Heart Association (AHA) reveals that college students who drink excessively can double their levels of C-reactive protein (CRP), a biological marker for inflammation that has been associated with a higher chance of cardiovascular problems. The 2007 AHA study asked 25 college students to complete surveys assessing lifestyle factors that put them at risk of increasing CRP levels, such as smoking, medication use and alcohol use.

For the record, heavy drinking was defined as three or more alcoholic drinks at least three days a week or at least five drinks two days a week. Compared with those of moderate drinkers (two to five drinks at a time, one or two days a week), the CRP levels of heavy drinkers were more than double, placing them in the zone associated with a moderate risk of heart disease.

It is not clear yet whether drinking heavily during your college years means you're setting yourself up for trouble down the line. To answer that, a long-term study would have to follow students once they entered middle age. Still, the concern is significant because enough studies already suggest a carry-over effect between past CRP levels and future heart disease.

Even so, becoming a teetotaler is not necessarily the pathway to ensuring a healthy heart in the future. This

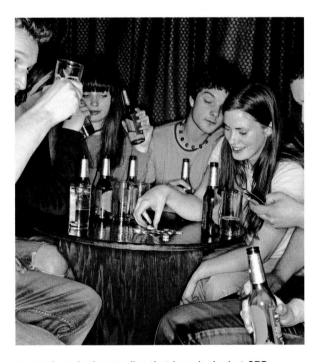

research and other studies that have looked at CRP levels in older populations found that nondrinkers (those who have one drink or less a week) actually have higher CRP numbers than those who drink in moderation. Somehow, moderate levels of alcohol may actually help protect against inflammation. And alcohol is known to reduce blood clotting. Red wine also contains additional beneficial chemicals, such as tannins, which slow atherosclerosis, and resveratrol, which has been shown to have anti-inflammatory effects.

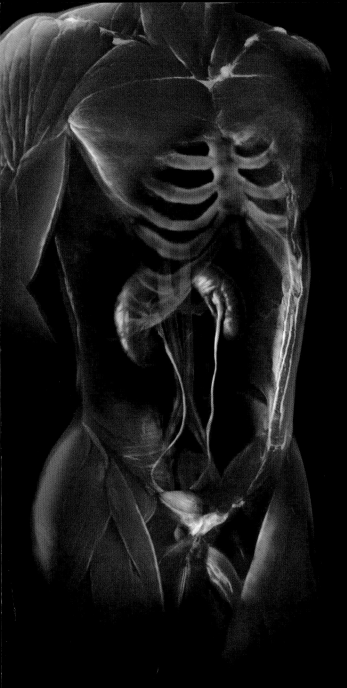

Every beat of your heart pushes blood under high pressure through your kidneys, a pair of bean-shaped organs, each the size of a clenched fist, that sit below the lungs on either side of the spine, just beneath your liver and spleen. Although the kidneys account for less than 1% of body weight, their work is so important and energy intensive that they absorb about 25% of the blood pumped out by the heart.

Within the kidneys, the blood vessels branch into tiny capillaries that further divide into microscopic filters called nephrons that pull impurities and waste products from the blood. The filtration process also isolates many nutrients and electrolytes we need to survive, but these are quickly cycled back into the bloodstream through reabsorption. More than 99% of the matter removed from our blood is selectively allowed back in, as the kidneys monitor and adjust the levels of water and salt in the body.

Waste matter that does not pass muster for reabsorption is mixed with water and passed down the ureters, a pair of 10-in.-long tubes that stretch to the urinary bladder, an inflatable sac within the pelvis. Muscle contractions ensure that this liquid, or urine, can move in only one direction, toward the bladder. Because the kidneys are constantly at work, a few drops of urine are passed into the bladder every 15 sec. or so, causing it to swell. A healthy adult bladder can hold up to 16 oz. of urine or more for several hours. As pressure builds, nerves within the bladder signal your brain that you are ready to urinate, and sphincter muscles at the base of the bladder (which prevent the expanding organ from leaking) relax. The urine passes from the bladder to the urethra and then out of the body.

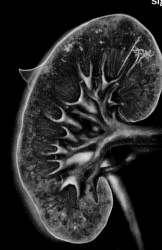

■ Briefing The Kidneys

Everything that comes in, must go out—one way or another. And the kidneys are where much of that transformation takes place in the human body. When protein is broken down during cellular digestion, it leaves behind urea in the bloodstream, a waste product that would be toxic if it were left to build up. When muscle cells reach the end of their life cycle and are replaced by new tissue, they throw off chemical debris known as creatinine. Normal metabolic processes also produce small amounts of chemicals such as ammonia. All of these must be removed—and quickly—before they damage tissues.

Blood filter *Above left and far right, the key organs of the urinary system inclue the kidneys, ureters, bladder and urethra. Above, the large renal artery feeds blood into the kidney*

Common Urinary Diseases and Disorders

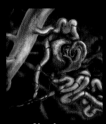

Nephron

Urinary Tract Infection

This common infection can affect the kidneys, ureters, urethra or bladder and is often caused by bacteria entering the urethra and migrating to the bladder, leading to inflammation and irritation in the lower urinary tract.

■ **Symptoms** *Cloudy or bloody urine; foul or strong odor; frequent or urgent need to urinate or need to urinate at night; pain or burning with urination; pressure in the lower pelvis.*

■ **Treatment** Mild cases may resolve quickly, but treatment is usually recommended to avoid the risk of infection spreading to the kidneys. In serious cases, antibiotics may be prescribed owing to the increased chance of deadly complications.

Kidney Failure
While the organs can deteriorate either quickly or more gradually, in both cases the kidneys lose their ability to remove waste and concentrate urine.

■ **Symptoms** *For acute, rapid failure: decrease in amount of urine or cessation of urination; excessive urination at night; fluid retention; swelling in the ankles, feet and legs; decreased sensation, especially in the hands or feet; metallic taste in mouth; persistent hiccups. For chronic, gradual failure: early symptoms include fatigue, frequent hiccups, general malaise, itching, headache,*

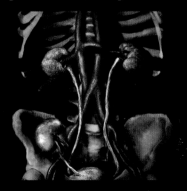

nausea, vomiting and unexpected weight loss. Later symptoms may include blood in vomit or in the stool, decreased alertness and frequent bruising or bleeding.

■ **Treatment** For acute cases: a hospital stay for dialysis, in which a machine takes on the filtering functions of an ailing kidney. For chronic cases: drugs to control symptoms, reduce complications and slow the progression of the disease. Dialysis or kidney transplantation may be required.

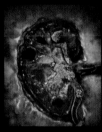

Crystals *Kidney stones (yellow) block urine flow*

Kidney Stones
Occur when a solid mass made up of tiny crystals forms within the kidneys and moves— painfully—down the ureter.

■ **Symptoms** *Abnormal urine color or blood in the urine; urinary pain, frequency, urgency or hesitancy in urination; pain in flank, back or groin.*

■ **Treatment** Kidney stones often pass on their own, and drugs can break down some forms. In severe cases, hospitalization may be needed to control symptoms or remove stones surgically or ultrasonically. Medicines and changing diet may prevent some types of stones from returning.

Urinary Incontinence
There are two types, stress and urge. Stress is an involuntary loss of urine during physical activity such as coughing, sneezing, standing or exercising. Urge is a strong, sudden need to urinate that can result in leakage.

■ **Symptoms** *Uncontrolled release of urine from the urethra.*

■ **Treatment** For stress: may include behavioral changes (including quitting smoking and changing diet), medication, pelvic floor muscle training and surgery. For urge: medication, bladder retraining, electrical stimulation and biofeedback therapy, and surgery.

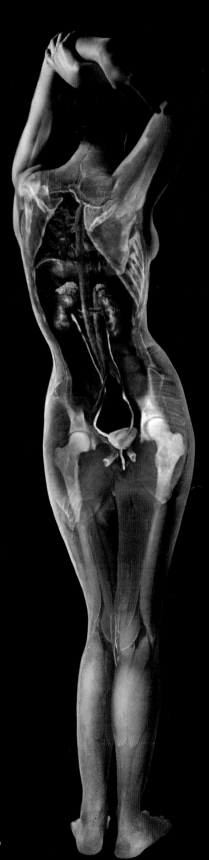

Three organs *Above, in this kidney transplant, the new organ is placed in the front quadrant of the abdomen, near major arteries, and the original kidneys are allowed to atrophy*

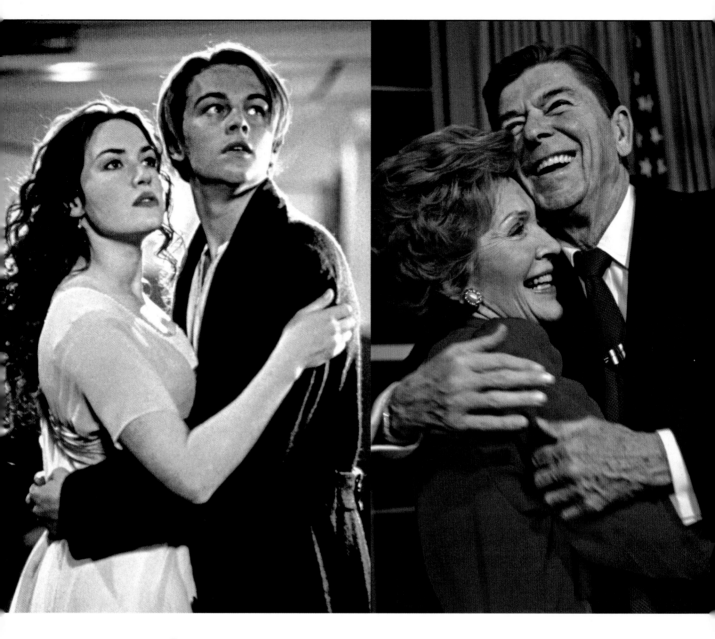

The Science of Romance

How our brains, bodies and senses help us fall in love

THE LAST TIME YOU HAD SEX, THERE WAS ARGUABLY not a thought in your head. O.K., if it was very familiar sex with a very familiar partner, the kind that—truth be told—you probably have most of the time, your mind may have wandered off to such decidedly nonerotic matters as balancing your checkbook. If it was the kind of sex you shouldn't have been having in the first place, you might have already been flashing ahead to the likely consequences. But if it was that kind of sex that's the whole reason you took up having sex in the first place—the out-of-breath, out-of-body, can-you-believe-this-is-actually-happening kind of sex—the rational you was very likely missing in action.

But mating and the rituals surrounding it make us come unhinged in other ways too, ones that are harder to explain by the mere babymaking imperative. There's the transcendent sense of tenderness you feel toward a person who sparks your interest. There's the sublime feeling of reward when that interest is returned; there are the flowers you buy and the poetry you write and the impulsive trip you make just so you can spend 48 hours in the presence of a lover. That's an awful lot of busy-work just to get a sperm to meet an egg—if merely getting a sperm to meet an egg is really all that it's about.

What scientists, not to mention the rest of us, want to know is, Why? What makes us go so loony over love?

70

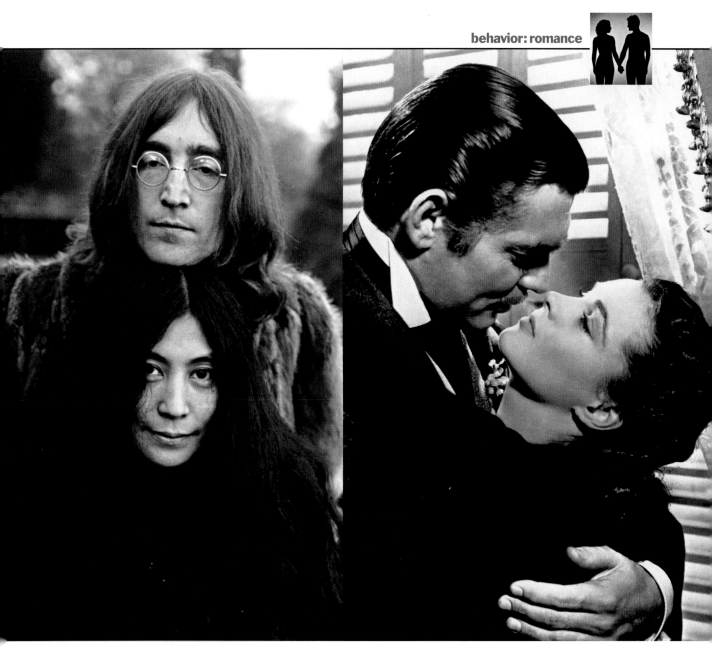

Four times two *From the movie screen to the popular song, love is often portrayed as an inexplicable urge, but scientists armed with new tools are dissecting the complex physiology behind romance*

Why would we bother with this elaborate exercise of fan dances and flirtations, winking and signaling, joy and sorrow? Today, our limited understanding is expanding. The more scientists look, the more they're able to tease romance apart into its individual strands—the visual, auditory, olfactory, tactile, neurochemical processes that make it possible. None of those things may be necessary for simple procreation, but all of them appear essential for something larger. What that something is—and how we achieve it— is only now coming clear.

If human reproductive behavior is a complicated thing, part of the reason is that it's designed to serve two clashing purposes. On the one hand, we're driven to mate a lot. On the other hand, we want to mate well so that our offspring survive. For that reason, no sooner do we reach sexual maturity than we learn to look for signals of good genes and reproductive fitness in potential partners and, significantly, to display them ourselves.

One of the most primal drivers of desire is that a possible partner smells right. Humans, like all animals, quickly learn to assign values to scents. Each human carries telltale smells of his or her own, and those can affect us in equally powerful ways. The best-known illustration of the invisible influence of scent is the way the menstrual cycles of women who live communally tend to synchronize. But how does one female signal the rest?

71

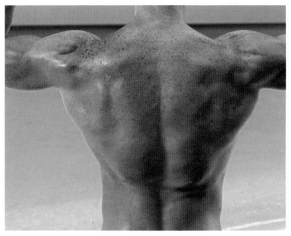

Women see broad shoulders as a sign of a man who can keep lions from the cave

The answer is almost certainly smell. Pheromones—or scent-signaling chemicals—are known to exist among animals, and while scientists have had a hard time unraveling the similar come-hither system in humans, they have isolated a few of the compounds. One type, known as driver pheromones, appears to affect the endocrine systems of others. Since the endocrine system plays a critical role in the timing of menstruation, there is at least a strong circumstantial case that the two are linked.

Scent may also help us narrow our choice of potential partners. Among the constellation of genes that control the immune system are those known as the major histocompatibility complex (MHC), which influence tissue rejection. Conceive a child with a person whose MHC is too similar to your own, and the risk of a miscarriage increases. Find a partner with sufficiently different MHC, and you're likelier to carry the baby to term. Recent studies show humans may be able to smell and taste MHC. Saliva contains the compound, which might explain the custom of kissing as a kind of taste test.

Less surprising than the importance of the way a partner smells is the way that partner looks and sounds. Humans are suckers for an attractive face and a sexy shape. Men see ample breasts and broad hips as indicators of a woman's ability to bear and nurse children—though most don't think about such matters so lucidly. Women see a broad chest and shoulders as a sign of someone who can be a capable provider, historically by clobbering a steady supply of meat and keeping lions away from the cave. A deep voice, also testosterone driven, can have similarly seductive power. Causation and mere correlation often get muddied in studies like this, but either way, a sexy voice at least appears to sell the goods.

If it's easy for a glance to become a kiss and a kiss to become much more, that's because your system is trip-wired to make it hard to turn back once you're aroused. That the kiss is the first snare is no accident. Kissing may serve the utilitarian purpose of providing a sample of MHC, but it also magnifies the other attraction signals—if only as a result of proximity. Scent is amplified up close, as are sounds and breaths and other cues. And none of that begins to touch the tactile experience that was entirely lacking until intimate contact was made.

Indeed, every kiss may also carry a chemical Mickey, slipped in by the male. Though testosterone is found in higher levels in men than in women, it is present in both genders and is critical in maintaining arousal states. Traces of testosterone make it into men's saliva, particularly among men who have high blood levels of the hormone to start with, and it's possible that a lot of kissing over a long period may be a way to pass some of that natural aphrodisiac to the woman, increasing her arousal and making her more receptive to even greater intimacy.

It's when the courting and kissing pay off—when you finally feel you've found the right person—that the true-love thrill hits, and studies of the brain with functional magnetic resonance imagers (fMRIs) show why it feels so good. The earliest fMRIs of brains in love were taken in 2000, and they revealed that the sensation of romance is processed in three areas. The first is the ventral tegmental, a clump of tissue in the brain's lower regions, which is the body's central refinery for dopamine. Dopamine does a lot of jobs, but the thing we notice most is that it regulates reward. When you win a hand of poker, it's a dopamine jolt that's responsible for the thrill. When you look forward to a big meal, it's the steady flow of dopamine that makes the anticipation such a pleasure.

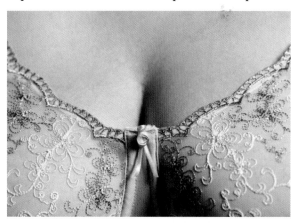

Men see ample breasts and broad hips as signs of a woman's fertility

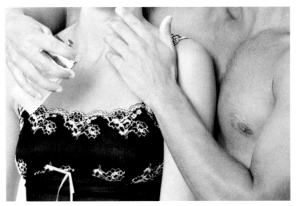

Scent may play an essential role in the process of finding a romantic partner

Anthropologist Helen Fisher at Rutgers University has conducted fMRI scans of people who are not just in love but newly in love and have found that their ventral tegmental areas are working particularly hard. "This little factory near the base of the brain is sending dopamine to higher regions," she says. "It creates craving, motivation, goal-oriented behavior—and ecstasy."

Even with its intoxicating supply of dopamine, the ventral tegmental couldn't do the love job on its own. Something has to turn the exhilaration of a new partner into what can approach an obsession, and that something is the brain's nucleus accumbens, located slightly higher and farther forward than the ventral tegmental. Thrill signals that start in the lower brain are processed in the nucleus accumbens via not just dopamine but also serotonin and, significantly, oxytocin.

If ever there was a substance designed to bind, it's oxy-

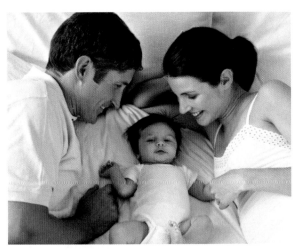

Men whose partners are pregnant experience elevated levels of oxytocin

tocin. New mothers are flooded with the stuff during labor and nursing—one reason they connect so ferociously to their babies before they know them as anything more than a squirmy body and a hungry mouth. Live-in fathers whose partners are pregnant experience elevated oxytocin too, a good thing if they're going to stick around through months of gestation and years of child-rearing.

The last major stops for love signals in the brain are the caudate nuclei, a pair of structures on either side of the head, each about the size of a shrimp. It's here that patterns and mundane habits, such as knowing how to type and drive a car, are stored. Motor skills like those can be hard to lose, thanks to the caudate nuclei's indelible memory. Apply the same permanence to love,

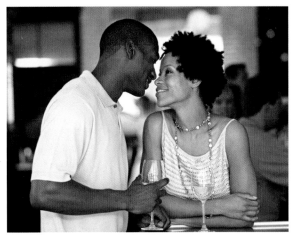

Kissing magnifies other basic signals of attraction: scent, sound and breath

and it's no wonder that early passion can gel so quickly into enduring commitment. The idea that even one primal part of the brain is involved in processing love would be enough to make the feeling powerful. The fact that three parts of the brain are at work processing love makes that powerful feeling consuming.

Survival of a species is a ruthless and reductionist matter, but if staying alive were truly all it was about, might we not have arrived at ways to do it without joy—as we could have developed language without literature, rhythm without song, movement without dance? Romance may be nothing more than reproductive filigree, a bit of decoration that makes us want to perpetuate the species and ensures that we do it right. But nothing could convince a person in love that there isn't something more at work—and the fact is, none of us would want to be convinced. That's a nut science may never fully crack. ∎

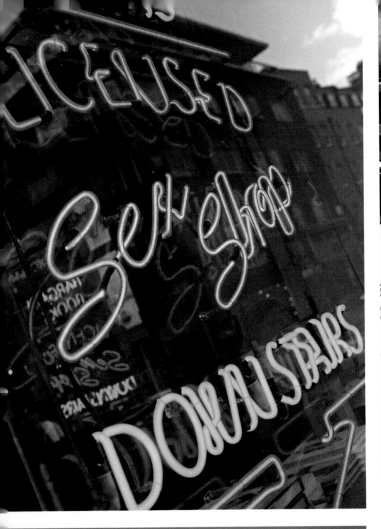
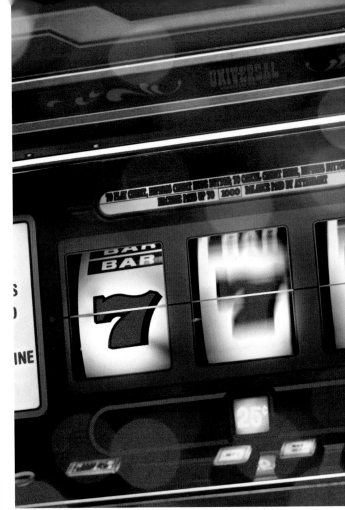
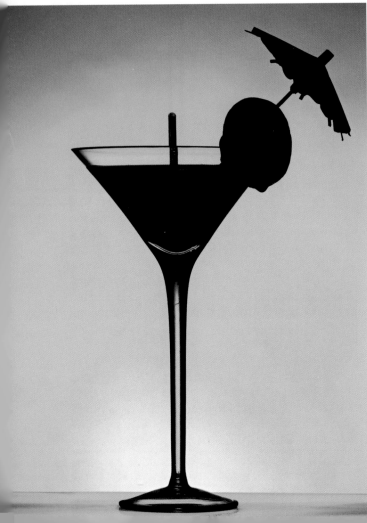
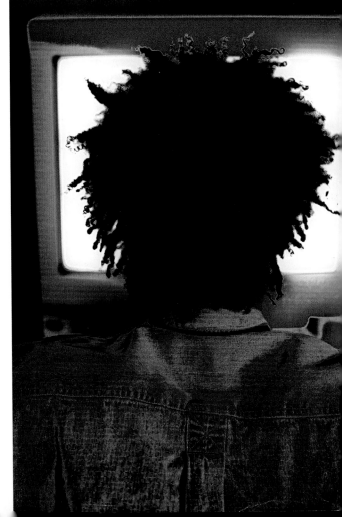

The Roots of Addiction

Brain research is discovering why we get hooked. Next, a cure?

THE BAD NEWS IS THAT ADDICTION TO HARMFUL SUB-
stances and behaviors continues to be a major
problem in the U.S. The good news: over the past
10 years, researchers have made real progress in understanding the physical basis of addiction. Armed with increasingly sophisticated technologies that chart mental
activity, investigators have begun to figure out exactly
what goes wrong in the brain of an addict—which neu-
rotransmitting chemicals are out of balance and what regions of the brain are affected. These scientists are developing a more detailed understanding of how deeply
and completely addiction can affect the brain, by hi-
jacking memory-making processes and by exploiting
emotions. And that's helped them design new drug treatments that are showing promise in cutting off the craving that drives an addict irresistibly toward relapse, a risk
faced by even the most dedicated abstainer.

"Addictions," says Joseph Frascella, director of the division of clinical neuroscience at the National Institute
on Drug Abuse (NIDA), "are repetitive behaviors in the
face of negative consequences, the desire to continue
something you know is bad for you." Addiction is such a
harmful behavior, in fact, that evolution should have
long ago weeded it out of the population: if it's hard to
drive safely under the influence, imagine trying to run
from a saber-toothed tiger or catch a squirrel for lunch.
And yet, says Dr. Nora Volkow, director of NIDA and a pioneer in the use of imaging to understand addiction, "the
use of drugs has been recorded since the beginning of
civilization. Humans in my view will always want to ex-
periment with things to make them feel good."

That's because drugs of abuse co-opt the very brain
functions that allowed our distant ancestors to survive in
a hostile world. Our minds are programmed to pay extra
attention to what neurologists call salience—that is, special relevance. Threats, for example, are highly salient,
which is why we instinctively try to get away from them.
But so are food and sex, because they help the individual
and the species survive. Drugs of abuse capitalize on this
ready-made programming. When exposed to drugs, our

Behaving badly *We think of addiction as an uncontrollable urge
for substances like alcohol and drugs, but behaviors such as gambling, sex, even cruising the Internet, can be addictive for some*

memory systems, reward circuits, decision-making skills
and conditioning kick in—salience in overdrive—to create an all-consuming pattern of uncontrollable craving.
"Some people have a genetic predisposition to addiction," says Volkow. "But because it involves these basic
brain functions, everyone will become an addict if sufficiently exposed to drugs or alcohol."

That can go for nonchemical addictions as well. Behaviors, from gambling to shopping to sex, may start out
as habits but slide into addictions. Sometimes there
might be a behavior-specific root of the problem. Volkow's research, for example, has shown that pathologi-
cally obese people who are compulsive eaters exhibit
hyperactivity in the areas of the brain that process food
stimuli from the mouth, lips and tongue. For such people, activating these regions is like opening the flood-
gates to the pleasure center. Almost anything deeply enjoyable can turn into an addiction, though.

Of course, not everyone becomes an addict. That's because we have other, more analytical regions that can

'Humans will always want to experiment with things to make them feel good.'
—Nora Volkow, director, NIDA

evaluate consequences and override mere pleasure seeking. Brain imaging is showing exactly how that happens.
Dr. Martin Paulus, a professor of psychiatry at the University of California at San Diego, looked at methamphetamine addicts enrolled in a VA hospital's intensive
four-week rehabilitation program. Those who were more
likely to relapse in the first year after completing the program were also less able to complete tasks involving cognitive skills and less able to adjust to new rules quickly.
This suggested that those patients might also be less
adept at using analytical areas of the brain while performing decision-making tasks.

Sure enough, brain scans showed that there were reduced levels of activation in the prefrontal cortex, where
rational thought can override impulsive behavior. It's
impossible to say if the drugs might have damaged these
abilities in the relapsers—an effect rather than a cause of
the chemical abuse—but the fact that the cognitive

deficit existed in only some of the meth users suggests that there was something innate that was unique to them. To his surprise, Paulus found that 80% to 90% of the time, he could accurately predict who would relapse within a year simply by examining the scans.

In their effort to decipher the physiological process of addiction, researchers are exploring the brain's reward system, powered largely by the neurotransmitter dopamine. They're focusing on the family of dopamine receptors that populate nerve cells and bind to the compound. The hope is that if you can dampen the effect of the brain chemical that carries the pleasure signal, you can loosen the drug's hold. For example, one particular group of dopamine receptors, called D3, seems to multi-

Shop till you drop *At least 1 in 20 Americans is a compulsive shopper, according to a Stanford University study. Defying stereotypes, the addiction affects both genders almost equally*

ply in the presence of cocaine, methamphetamine and nicotine, making it possible for more of the drug to enter and activate nerve cells.

If dopamine receptors are the gas, the brain's own inhibitory systems act as the brakes. But in addicts, this natural damping circuit, called GABA (gamma-amino-butyric acid), appears to be faulty, so the brain never appreciates that it has been satiated. Enter vigabatrin, an antiepilepsy drug marketed in 60 countries (but not yet in the U.S.). An effective GABA booster, vigabatrin helps epileptics suppress overactive motor neurons that can

cause muscles to go into spasm. Suspecting that enhancing the GABA levels in addicts' brains might help them control their drug cravings, two U.S. biotech firms are studying vigabatrin's effect on methamphetamine and cocaine users. So far, in animals, vigabatrin prevents the breakdown of GABA so that more of the inhibitory compound can be stored in whole form in nerve cells. That way, more of it could be released when those cells are activated by a hit from a drug. Because it targets the brain's global suppression system, researchers hope vigabatrin may be effective against all forms of addiction.

Another important discovery: evidence is building to support the 90-day rehabilitation model, which is used by Alcoholics Anonymous (new AA members are urged to attend daily meetings for their first 90 days) and is the length of most stints in drug-treatment programs. It turns out that this is just about how long it takes for the brain to reset itself and shake off the immediate influence of a drug. Researchers at Yale University have documented what they call the sleeper effect—a gradual re-engaging of proper decision making and analytical functions in the brain's prefrontal cortex— after an addict has abstained for at least 90 days.

This work has led to research on cognitive enhancers, or compounds that may amplify connections in the prefrontal cortex to speed up the natural reversal. Such enhancement would give the higher regions of the brain a fighting chance against the amygdala, a more basal region that plays a role in priming the dopamine-reward system when certain cues suggest imminent pleasure— anything from the sight of white powder that looks like cocaine to spending time with friends you used to drink with. It's that conditioned reflex that unleashes a craving.

With increasing certainty, scientists say that extinguishing urges is not simply a matter of getting one's cravings for substances or behavior to fade but of helping the addict learn a new form of conditioning, a sort of rewiring that allows the brain's cognitive power to shout down the amygdala and other lower regions. Or, as recovering AA members like to say, "Recovery is a process, not an event; it takes time." ■

Substance and Behavioral Addictions

Addicted America

Drugs An estimated **3.6 million** people are dependent on drugs. Each day some 8,000 people try them for the first time; 700,000 more are being treated for addiction. Cocaine, marijuana and prescription pain relievers are the most abused.

Tobacco There are about **71.5 million** users of tobacco products in the U.S. Some **23.4%** of men and **18.5%** of women are cigarette smokers, with cigarette use lowest in Western states and highest in the Midwest; 44.3% of young adults ages 18 to 25 use tobacco, the highest rate for any age group.

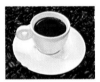

Caffeine It's the most widely used mood-altering drug in the world and is routinely ingested by about **80% to 90%** of Americans, primarily through soda and coffee. A daily brewed cup of joe, with 100 mg of caffeine, can lead to physical dependence. Withdrawal symptoms are experienced by **40% to 70%** of those trying to stop.

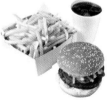

Food An addiction to food affects as many as **4 million** U.S. adults and is strongly linked to depression. About 15% of mildly obese people are compulsive eaters. Binge eating, thought to be the most common eating disorder in America, is considered bulimia when a person purges to lose weight.

What happens in the brain

1. We feel good when neurons in the reward pathway release a neurotransmitter called dopamine into the nucleus accumbens and other brain areas.

2. Neurons in the reward pathway communicate by sending electrical signals down their axons. The signal is passed to the next neuron across a small gap called the synapse.

3. Dopamine is released into the synapse, crosses to the next neuron and binds to receptors, providing a jolt of pleasure. Excess dopamine is taken back up by the sending cell. Other nerve cells release GABA, an inhibitory neurotransmitter that works to prevent the receptor nerve from being overstimulated.

4. Addictive substances increase the amount of dopamine in the synapse, heightening the feeling of pleasure. Addiction occurs when repeated drug use disrupts the normal balance of brain circuits that control rewards, memory and cognition, ultimately leading to compulsive drug taking.

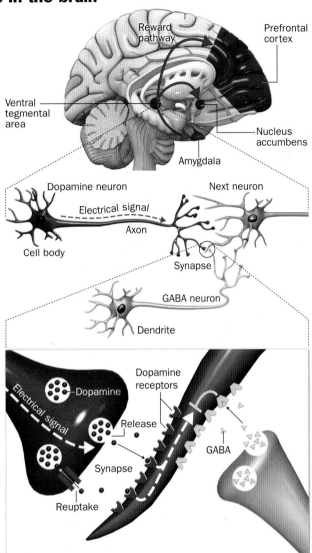

Reward pathway — Prefrontal cortex — Ventral tegmental area — Nucleus accumbens — Amygdala

Dopamine neuron — Next neuron — Electrical signal — Axon — Cell body — Synapse — GABA neuron — Dendrite

Electrical signal — Dopamine — Dopamine receptors — Release — GABA — Synapse — Reuptake

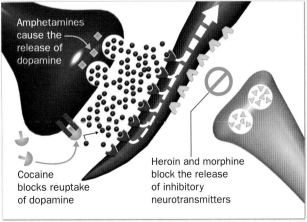

Amphetamines cause the release of dopamine — Cocaine blocks reuptake of dopamine — Heroin and morphine block the release of inhibitory neurotransmitters

Source: National Institute on Drug Abuse (NIH)
TIME Diagram by Kristina Dell, Meg Massey and Joe Lertola

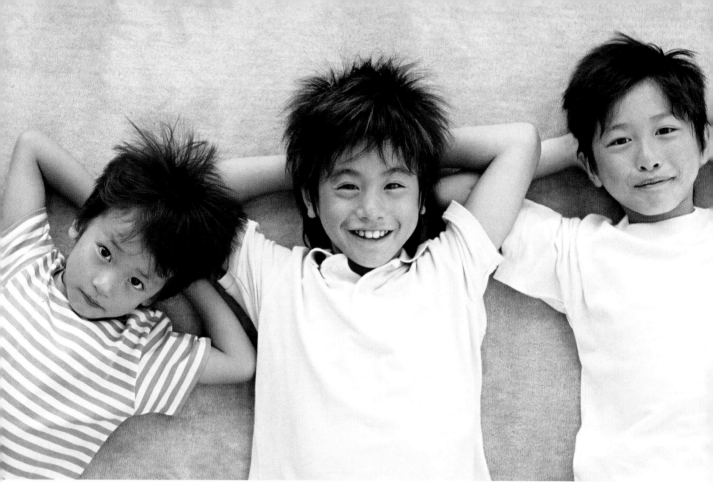

The Secrets of Birth Order

Where you end up may depend on where you started from

LIFE DEALT ELLIOTT ROOSEVELT A TOUGH HAND. IF the alcohol wasn't getting him, the morphine was. If it wasn't the morphine, it was the struggle with depression. Then, of course, there were the constant comparisons with big brother Teddy—all of which culminated when Elliott died of alcoholism at 34. Seven years later, Teddy became President at 42.

Elliott Roosevelt was not the only younger sibling of an eventual President to cause his family headaches. There was Donald Nixon, Billy Carter and Roger Clinton, each a problem to his Oval Office elder. And there is Neil Bush, younger sib of both a President and a Governor, implicated in the savings-and-loan scandals of the 1980s, who lamented to his estranged wife in a 2002 letter, "I've lost patience for being compared to my brothers."

Welcome to a very big club, Bro. Of all the things that shape who we are, few seem more arbitrary than the sequence in which we and our siblings pop out of the womb. Yet in family after family, case study after case study, the simple roll of the birth-date dice has an odd and arbitrary power all its own.

The importance of birth order has been known—or at least suspected—for years. But increasingly, there's hard evidence of its impact. In June 2007, a group of Norwe-

gian researchers released a study showing that firstborns are generally smarter than any siblings who come along later, enjoying on average a three-point IQ advantage over the next eldest—probably a result of the intellectual boost that comes from mentoring younger siblings and helping them in day-to-day tasks. The second child, in turn, is a point ahead of the third.

The differences don't stop there. Studies in the Philippines show that later-born siblings tend to be shorter and weigh less than earlier-borns. Younger siblings are less likely to be vaccinated than older ones, with last-borns getting immunized sometimes at only half the rate of firstborns. Eldest siblings are also disproportionately represented in high-paying professions. Younger siblings, by contrast, are looser cannons, less educated and less strapping, perhaps, but statistically likelier to live the exhilarating life of an artist or a comedian, an adventurer, entrepreneur, GI or firefighter. And middle children? Well, they can be a puzzle—even to birth-order researchers.

Firstborns do more than survive; they thrive. A 2007 survey of corporate heads conducted by Vistage, an international organization of CEOs, found that 43% of the people who occupy the big chair in boardrooms are firstborns, 33% are middle-borns, and 23% are last-borns. Eldest siblings are disproportionately represented among surgeons and M.B.A.s too, according to Stanford University psychologist Robert Zajonc.

At the other end of the family spectrum, younger siblings struggle early on to shake up the existing order, often with subversive humor. Families abound with stories of last-borns who are the clowns of the brood, able to get their way simply by being funny or outrageous. Some of history's great satirists—Voltaire, Jonathan Swift, Mark Twain—were among the youngest members of large families, a pattern that continues today. Faux bloviator Stephen Colbert often points out that he's the last of 11 children.

Personality tests show that while firstborns score especially well on the dimension of temperament known as conscientiousness—a sense of general responsibility and follow-through—later-borns score higher on what's known as agreeableness, or the simple ability to get along in the world. Later-borns, however, don't try merely to please other people; they also try to provoke them. Later-borns are similarly willing take risks with their physical safety, the likeliest to choose the kind of activities that could cause injury.

If eldest sibs are the dogged achievers and youngest sibs are the gamblers and comics, where does this leave those in between? That it's so hard to define what middle-borns may become is due to their constantly evolving role in the family dynamic. Unlike the firstborn, who spends at least some time as the only-child eldest, and the last-born, who hangs around long enough to become the only-child youngest, middlings are never alone and thus never get 100% of the parents' investment of time and money. The youngest in the family, but only until someone else comes along, they are both teacher and student, babysitter and babysat, too young for the privileges of the firstborn but too old for the latitude given the last. Stuck for life in a center seat, middle children get shortchanged, even on family resources.

But can your place in the family really play such a strong role in who you become? Birth order, of course, is only one of countless factors that influence our lives. The most vocal detractors of birth-order research question less the findings of the science than the methods. Families, they point out, are very different things—distinguished by size, income, hometown, education, religion, ethnicity and more—so it's hard to reduce them to statistics. True enough. Yet millenniums of families would swear by the power of birth order to shape the adults we eventually become. ∎

Siblings and Rivals Every birdie in the nest can't be equal

For every famous sibling, there are often a few others in the brood who might like the spotlight too. Some get it; some don't; some wish they hadn't. Few find the competition easy.

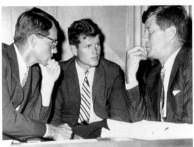

The Kennedys Father Joe would pit his four sons against one another in sports, education and achievement, leading to both tragedy and triumph. When Joe Jr. died in World War II, younger brother John picked up the torch of his father's dreams.

The Jacksons Michael, the youngest of the five brothers in the Jackson 5, showed a late child's desire for the spotlight and ability to please. The only member of the family to come close to his solo stardom was the youngest of 9 children, sister Janet. The oldest sibling, sister Rebbie, had to sing backup.

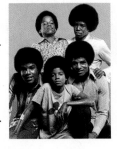

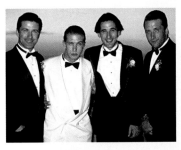

The Baldwins Alec, left, is the senior member of this acting clan, which includes Stephen, William and Daniel. Sisters Jane and Elizabeth avoided show biz. As Wikipedia notes, reinforcing the birth-order hypothesis, Alec "is the oldest and most famous of the Baldwin brothers."

The Williamses No rivalry in sports can match the long-running duel between sisters Venus, left, and Serena Williams, who faced each other in the Wimbledon final in 2008, right, with elder sister Venus winning the match. The two have now faced off seven times in the final of a major tournament.

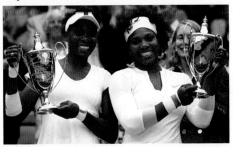

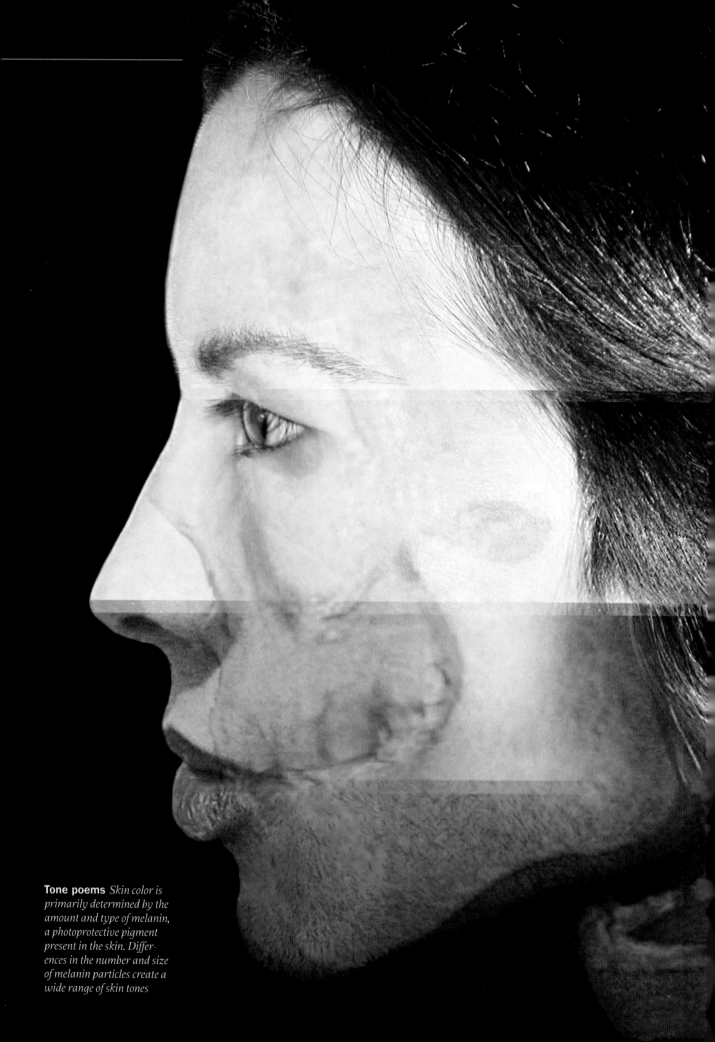

Tone poems *Skin color is primarily determined by the amount and type of melanin, a photoprotective pigment present in the skin. Differences in the number and size of melanin particles create a wide range of skin tones*

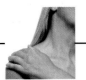

Preserve and Protect

A membrane of skin: the inside story on our outside layer

THINK OF WHAT THE WALLS AND ROOF OF YOUR home do: they warm you in winter and cool you in summer. They keep out the elements and would-be intruders while also defining a boundary between your inner sanctum and the outer world. Your skin, the largest (and in some ways the most complex) organ in your body, does all of this and more.

Like your home, one of skin's primary functions is to preserve and to protect. So while four of the human senses are housed in specific parts of the body, our capacity to detect that we are being touched and to distinguish between various temperatures, pressures and levels of pain resides everywhere at once, thanks to the skin.

Making up about 15% of your total body mass, the skin weighs around 10 lbs. in an average adult, and it takes up an area of approximately 20 sq. ft., roughly the size of a twin-bed sheet. Each square inch contains thousands of cells, along with hundreds of blood vessels and nerve endings, plus hundreds of lymph vessels and glands for producing sweat, oil and hair. Your skin also takes in nutrients. It manufactures vitamin D with an assist from the sun's ultraviolet radiation, which helps with bone maintenance and repair. And it expels excess water and electrolytes, along with waste nitrogen, from the body.

Don't be deceived, however: the wrapping you actually see in the mirror does none of these things. The outermost layer of skin, called the epidermis, consists entirely of dead cells. This used-up tissue falls away from your body at the rate of 30,000 cells per minute (that's almost 50 million per day), and it is responsible for much of the dust you find in your home. Every month or so, you are wrapped in entirely new skin, and over the course of a lifetime, you will shed almost 20 lbs. of epidermis.

The layer below, called the dermis, is a bit more active: packed with living tissue and humming metabolic activity, this section of your skin also contains two crucial proteins: collagen, which gives skin strength, and elastin, which enables skin to stretch and then return to its original shape.

Human skin is unique among animal integuments in several ways. As Nina Jablonski, an anthropologist at Pennsylvania State University and author of *Skin: A Natural History*, points out, it follows a "naked/sweaty" model that trades the furry coat common among other mammals for a prodigious capacity to cool off through perspiration.

In contrast to humans with skin that perspires, many mammalian species must limit strenuous physical activity to short, intense bursts to avoid overheating. The panting of a winded dog illustrates this alternate form of cooling. A dog's circulatory system rushes warm blood from its interior to the tongue, which has a large surface area, is exposed to air and is covered with moist saliva. The resulting evaporation cools the blood, which is then rushed back into the body's warm interior, helping to reduce its internal temperature. Elephants and cows cool off using the same mechanism.

The outermost layer of the skin is not alive; it is made up of dead cells, which are constantly falling away. Over your lifetime, your body will shed almost 20 lbs. of dead skin

Human skin acts as a natural HVAC unit in other ways too. When body temperature spikes, the circulatory vessels in the skin open to increase blood flow to the surface, cooling it down; that's why skin appears flushed when we are overheated. When the air outside the skin is too cold, however, vessels in the skin contract, reducing the flow of blood to the surface and fighting heat loss; that's why the skin often appears pale, or even blue, when we are cold.

When our skin isn't changing color due to the temperature, it's the amount of melanin it contains that determines its tone. Our personal skin color is part of what makes us human: as Jablonski also points out, humans are unusual among animals in the range of natural skin colors we display within a single species—a gorgeous mosaic indeed. ■

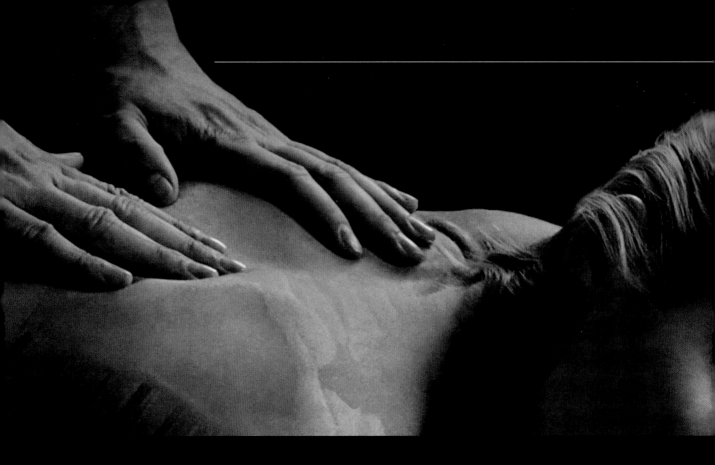

■ Anatomy Lesson The Integumentary System

The skin is part of what anatomists call the "integumentary system," which includes the hair and nails. In most areas, the skin is about the thickness of a few sheets of paper, but it reaches its greatest width, about 15/100 of an inch, on the palms of the hands and soles of the feet, which require extra padding. It is thinnest (roughly 2/100 of an inch) on the eyelids and scalp.

Many biologists now classify a membrane that separates a living thing from its environment as one of the three defining characteristics of life, along with a metabolism to produce energy and a genetic code to make copies of itself. For human beings, skin is that membrane. Humans need water to thrive, and the skin functions as a waterproof sack that enables us to carry within us the moisture we need to survive. Skin also plays a crucial role in keeping bacteria and parasites from accessing our other organs.

While all skin tissue is sensitive to touch, certain areas—especially the hands, fingertips, eyelids, genitals, lips and tongue—contain two types of specialized receptors, Meissner's corpuscles and Merkel's discs, which can detect even the faintest pressure. Other specialized receptors sense pain and temperature, but they are not distributed evenly. An average square inch of skin surface contains some 1,200 pain receptors but only about 100 receptors for pressure, 40 for cold and six for warmth.

The skin of the epidermis is rich in a protein called

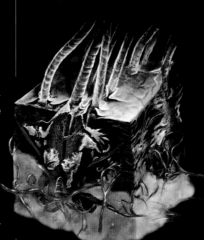

Skin deep *Three layers of skin: the thin top layer, or epidermis (light color), consists of dead cells ready to be shed. The thicker dermis beneath (brown) is the anchor for hair follicles (purple) and holds sweat and oil glands, blood vessels and sensory receptors (red). The subcutaneous layer, or hypodermis (yellow), consists mainly of fat, which nourishes and insulates the dermis*

sue that sprout from the skin: hair and nails. Although we have less hair than our mammalian cousins, our entire body is nearly covered with it—everywhere except our lips, nipples, the soles of our feet and the palms of our hands. Hair is composed almost entirely of keratin, but the only part of it that is alive is the root, buried deep within the dermis. All the hair we can see is dead tissue. Our finger- and toenails are also composed of keratin, packed densely in flat sheets. Like bone tissue, human nails are stronger than granite of the same

Common Skin Diseases and Disorders

Acne Condition caused by clogged pores that form whiteheads, blackheads or inflamed red pimples, most commonly on the face and shoulders but sometimes appearing on the trunk, arms, legs and buttocks.

■ **Symptoms** *Eruptions with inflammation and/or redness on the surrounding skin, cysts, pustules, scarring of the skin and whiteheads.*

■ **Treatment** Cleaning the skin and hair and avoiding squeezing or scratching pimples can lessen the effects. Over-the-counter acne medications can help by killing bacteria, drying up oil and causing skin to peel. Prescription medicines include oral antibiotics, topical antibiotics, retinoic acid cream or gel (Retin-A) and isotretinoin pills.

Eczema Also called dermatitis, this is a term for several different types of swelling that are not dangerous but cause red, swollen and itchy skin.

■ **Symptoms** *Blisters with oozing and crusting; dry, leathery skin areas; ear discharge or bleeding; intense itching; rash, redness and inflammation.*

■ **Treatment** Soothing moisturizers, mild soaps, or wet dressings; topical corticosteroids (low potency); ointments or creams that contain tar compounds; anti-inflammatory medicines.

Male Pattern Baldness Hair loss due to shrinkage of follicles caused by hormones and genetic predisposition.

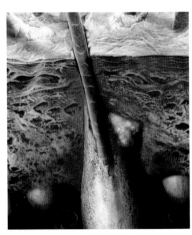

Follicle *Hairs are rooted in these bulbous roots within the scalp or skin*

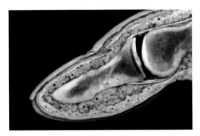

Digit *Cutaway view of index finger shows layers of dermis around bone*

■ **Symptoms** *The typical pattern is a receding hairline and hair thinning.*

■ **Treatment** Drugs include minoxidil (Rogaine) and finasteride (Propecia); hair transplants via plugs.

Melanoma Skin cancer that afflicts pigment cells, or melanocytes, making them malignant.

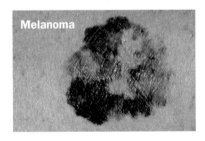
Melanoma

■ **Symptoms** *Most often, a change in the size, shape, color or feel of an existing skin mole.*

■ **Treatment** Minor surgery to remove the tumor; radiation or laser therapy.

Psoriasis A buildup of dead cells on the skin's surface, leading to redness and irritation. Cause is unknown, but may occur when the body's immune system mistakes healthy cells for foreign substances.

■ **Symptoms** *Irritated patches of skin, most often on the elbows, knees and trunk. Additional symptoms may include genital lesions in males; joint pain or aching; nail thickening, spots or dents on the nail surface.*

■ **Treatment** Cortisone cream, moisturizers and prescription medicines containing vitamin D or vitamin A (retinoids). Severe cases may be treated with drugs to suppress the body's immune response.

Source: National Institutes of Health

By the Numbers
Skin, Hair & Nails

5,000,000
Number of individual hairs on the average adult human body

100,000
Number of hairs on the average adult scalp

30,000
Number of dead epidermal cells that your body sheds—each minute

90 ft.
Total length of the fingernails grown by a human over the course of an average lifetime

25-45 days
Time it takes for all the epidermal skin on your body to be shed and replaced

20 sq. ft.
Total area of your skin, rolled flat, should Dr. Hannibal Lecter take a fancy to you

20 lbs.
Total weight of the dead skin your body will shed over the course of a lifetime

10 lbs.
Total weight of the skin, hair and nails on the average adult body

4 x
Speed at which our fingernails grow faster than our toenails

■On the Horizon Briefs

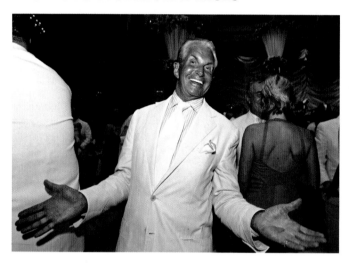

Should You Run from the Sun? Here's the latest on skin care and solar rays

We can't all tan like George Hamilton, above, but far too many of us are trying—and frying. The quandary: excessive exposure to ultraviolet (UV) radiation causes skin cancer, premature aging and cataracts, but we also need a little ray of sunshine or two to help keep our bones strong. So here's a Q&A on having fun in the sun, safely:

Does sun exposure increase the body's level of vitamin D?
Yes. The body uses UV light to make vitamin D, which is vital for bone health, but the fair-skinned need only a few minutes of summer-sun exposure and can get their winter D from fortified milk or vitamins.

Is indoor tanning any safer than sunbathing?
No. UV lamps come with all the health risks of natural sunlight. They emit some vitamin-D-inducing UVB rays, which in excess cause sunburns and skin cancer, and many more UVA rays, which cause wrinkles and can lead to skin cancer.

How much protection does sunscreen offer?
A lot, when used properly. That entails slathering on a shot glass's worth every two hours, regardless of whether the lotion is touted as waterproof, sweatproof or has a high SPF (sun-protection factor). SPF refers to the ability to deflect burning UVB rays (SPF 15 deflects 93% of them; SPF 30 blocks 97%), but it says nothing about protection from UVA rays, which are just as harmful. Look for broad-spectrum sunscreens that contain Parsol 1789, zinc oxide, titanium dioxide or Mexoryl. And reapply often, even on cloudy days.

Are spray-on tans and sunless tanning lotions safe?
Mostly. Many dermatologists are recommending them to patients who want to look tan. The active ingredient, dihydroxyacetone, affects only the outermost layer of skin and fades with exfoliation. One cautionary note: use these products in conjunction with sunscreen.

Should those with naturally dark skin worry about the sun?
Yes. The melanin in black and brown skin offers only partial protection from UV rays, not unlike a base tan. Although melanoma is far more common among whites, it is more likely to be fatal among blacks and Hispanics because the cancer progresses longer undetected.

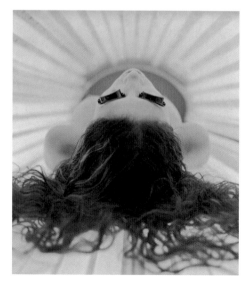

Tanning, Teens, Trouble They cook hot to look hot—but skin cancer in kids is exploding

Every year some 2.3 million teens pop into a tanning parlor, helping make indoor tanning a $5 billion-a-year business. Dermatologists, however, are alarmed by the risks of so much exposure to ultraviolet (UV) radiation. Easy access to insta-tans, doctors say, may be driving a frightening spike in skin-cancer rates among the young. The incidence of melanoma, the most lethal form of skin cancer, has doubled in the U.S. since 1975 among women ages 15 to 29. The World Health Organization estimated in 2006 that as many as 60,000 deaths world-wide are caused each year by excessive UV exposure and urged youths under 18 to steer clear of indoor tanning.

Looking for ways to enforce this recommendation, some U.S. states have prohibited youngsters under 14 from using tanning parlors. The larger challenge involves changing the adolescent culture that encourages tanning. Meanwhile, some new research indicates that tanning may release endorphins and, like nicotine, may be addicting.

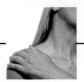

The Skinny on Skin Care Lotions, potions and notions: a roundup of new trends in treatment

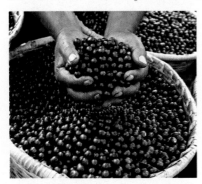

Acai berries *Exposure to strong sunlight helps them resist harmful UV rays*

Like the rest of us, cosmetics makers are going green, releasing a host of new skin lotions and treatments that draw on exotic natural plants—and a few familiar old faces liberated from the liquor cabinet—for their potency. Here are a few among the brave new world of skin treatments that claim to bring you both beauty and good health.

Acai Berries Antioxidants, commonly found in fruits and vegetables, are the body's defense against free radicals—reactive chemicals that are needed to destroy viruses and bacteria but can be harmful to healthy cells. Fast-acting radicals are the hardest to scavenge, and to help our bodies out, cosmetics companies are turning to a berry from the Amazon, acai, which in tests proved better at hunting down free radicals than nearly any other fruit. Why? The palm trees that sprout the acai berries occupy the canopy at the very top of the rain forest. So their berries are strongly exposed to ultraviolet radiation and have had to develop chemical strategies to deal with it, making them a valuable resource for skin health.

Arctic Berries Sea buckthorn berry oil is a popular home remedy for scrapes and burns in Russia and Nordic countries. Now sea buckthorn and 10 or so other berries that grow in Arctic regions, including Arctic raspberry, cloudberry and cowberry, are the miracle medicine du jour, thanks to their supply of essential fatty acids (EFAs) and antioxidants. More than just maintaining and moist-

urizing the lipid-rich epidermis, EFAs work to lighten skin tone, diminish age spots and reduce inflammation.

Glacial Facials After a trip to Iceland in 2004, cosmetics executive Sarah Kugelman was so inspired by the purity and richness of the remote country's glacial waters, medicinal botanicals and nutrient-packed plants that she decided to find a way to bottle that bounty and bring back a little bit of Iceland for everyone. Result: Skyn Iceland, named after the Icelandic word for "senses." All its products contain what she calls a unique blend of Iceland's mineral-laden glacial waters (which Kugelman imports), botanical herbs and anti-oxidant-rich plants. More ingredients

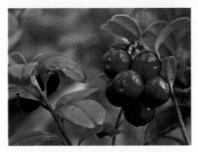

Cowberry *These Nordic beauties are rich in antioxidants and fatty acids*

address specific skin needs. *Angelica archangelica,* for instance, an herb in the brand's night cream and healing serum that is related to ginseng, aids the immune system in warding off infections. Cloudberry-seed oil, which contains moisturizing fatty acids, is included in the daily face lotion, while

Red wine *From the dinner table to the spa*

the antistress oral spray, spritzed under the tongue, boasts theanine from green tea, which helps the body relax.

Red Wine It has long been known that a glass of red wine is good for you, but now health spas are using it in their treatments. In South Africa, "vino-therapy" clients are massaged and bathed in wine and vine extracts. Supporters insist that grape antioxidants are more powerful than vitamins C and E, help restore elasticity in the skin, improve circulation and combat premature aging. Result: wine baths that wash the body with grape seeds, skins, stalks and pulp, while the epidermis is scrubbed with essential oils and crushed seeds from grapes. In the merlot and Chardonnay wraps, you're plastered in a grape paste, wrapped in plastic and lowered onto a waterbed. And to think some folks still buy wine to drink!

Sake Japan's sake brewers are releasing skin-care lines featuring their rice wines. With high levels of naturally created amino acids, these New Age elixirs are aimed at moisturizing and protecting the skin without irritation. The inspiration: geishas once applied sake to their faces before putting on makeup, and the nation's *toji* (head brewers) have long been famed for their soft hands.

Sake *It's not just for drinking anymore, say Japan's rice-wine brewers*

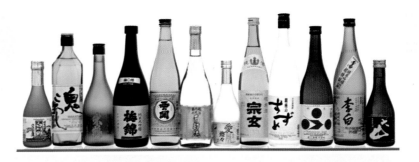

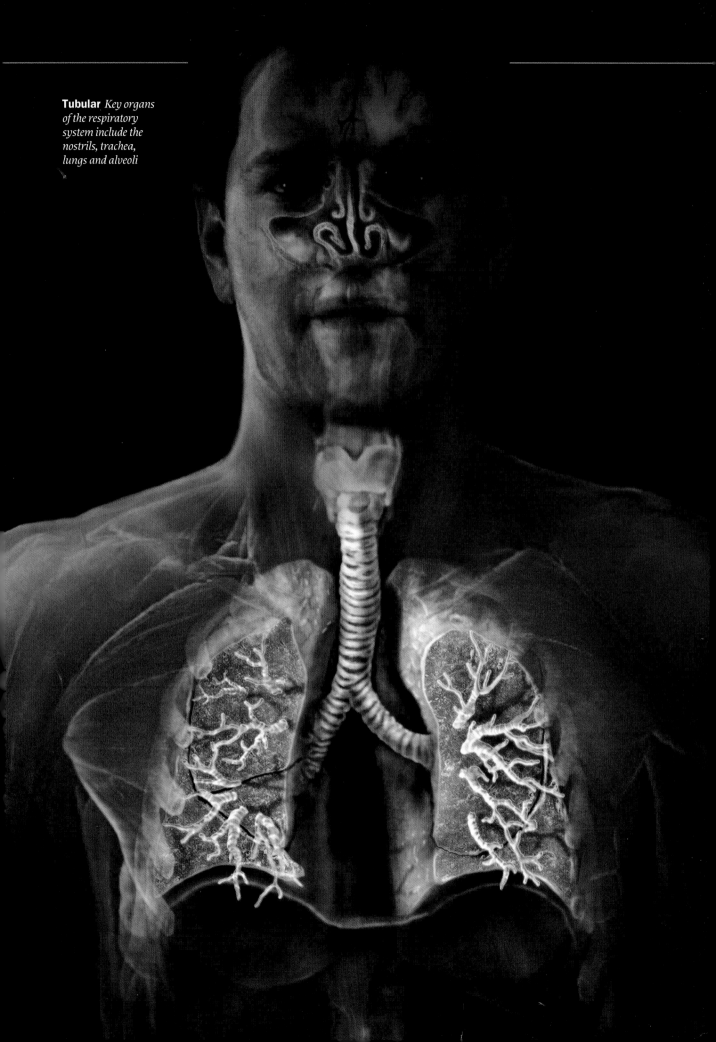

Tubular *Key organs of the respiratory system include the nostrils, trachea, lungs and alveoli*

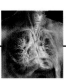

United Air Lines

What a gas! Oxygen, carbon dioxide, the lungs and breathing

EVERY BREATH YOU TAKE IS AN ELABORATELY CHOREographed ballet of chemistry and body mechanics. Between 15 and 20 times each minute, and more often in moments of heavy exertion, the diaphragm, a horizontal wall of muscle above your abdomen, contracts and pulls the bottom of your lungs downward. At the same time, the sheet of intercostal muscles woven between your ribs tugs the upper section of your lungs upward and outward. This stretching causes the elastic, spongy tissue of your lungs to expand, which drops the pressure of the gases inside. Yet nature abhors even a partial vacuum, so air rushes in through your nasal passages and mouth and raises the pressure inside your lungs once more.

A few seconds later, your diaphragm and intercostal muscles relax, your lungs contract, and the air pressure inside goes up. This higher pressure causes air to rush out through the nose and mouth. In the course of an average day, you will repeat this cycle more than 20,000 times, taking in and pushing out more than 5,000 gal. of air.

This external respiration is only the most obvious of the three steps of breathing. In the next process, internal respiration, incoming air is funneled through an elaborate, branching network of lung passages and filtered down into more than 300 million microscopic sacs, or alveoli, each one of which is surrounded by equally minute blood vessels, or capillaries. Here, oxygen is harvested from air breathed in, or "inspired," a moment earlier and passed through the walls of both alveoli and capillaries, then attached to red blood cells to be carried throughout the body. At the same time, carbon dioxide (CO_2) is passed back from the capillaries to the alveoli, to be expelled when we breathe out, or "expire."

Finally, there is cellular respiration, as oxygen-rich blood travels from the lungs to all living tissue in the body, where the exchange process that took place within the lungs is repeated at the cellular level, and the oxygenated blood is traded for CO_2.

The air we breathe in is more like the gas we push out of our lungs than you might think. Incoming air contains about 20% oxygen, with less than 1% CO_2 and water vapor; the rest is nitrogen, trace gases and particulate matter. The air we exhale is still about 16% oxygen but now contains around 4% CO2 and 6% water vapor. This high oxygen content explains why the life-saving technique of mouth-to-mouth resuscitation actually works, rather than suffocating the person in distress.

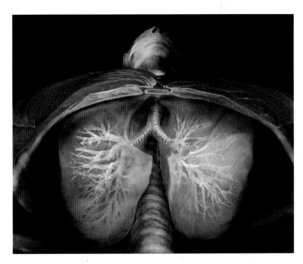

Bellows *The larger tubes through which air flows into the lungs are bronchi, which branch into smaller tubes called bronchioles. When these pathways reach their smallest size, they are called alveoli*

Specialized cells called chemoreceptors constantly monitor oxygen and carbon dioxide levels in the blood, then signal the brain to speed up or slow down the respiration rate. Our breathing is so efficient that we usually make use of only about one-fifth of the lungs' capacity to process air. A final wonder: air that enters our body through the mouth or nostrils is heated or cooled to within three degrees or so of body temperature by the time it reaches the lungs, regardless of how hot or cold it was when first inspired, a second or less earlier. ∎

Anatomy Lesson The Respiratory System

Your respiratory system looks something like an upside-down tree, the base of which is rooted in your head. That's where the mouth and nasal passages take in air, filtering, warming and humidifying it. They pass it to the pharynx, where the two routes converge. Air then blows through the larynx, or voice box, which houses the vocal cords, where a mucous lining filters out some impurities. Next, the air moves down the trachea, or windpipe, which makes up the trunk of our respiratory tree. It is lined with microscopic hairs called cilia that filter out more impurities and pass them back toward the throat, where they can be swallowed or expelled through coughing. Air then flows into one of the two bronchi, which lead left and right into our two lungs. These are separated by a structure called the mediastinum, which houses the heart, trachea, esophagus and several major blood vessels. The lungs take up most of the chest cavity, filling the space inside the ribs above the diaphragm and below the collarbone. Surprisingly, these air organs are not created equal: the left lung is slightly smaller than the right, to make room for the heart, which nestles just left of center within the chest, and the stomach, which sits higher on the body's left side than on the right. For this reason, the right lung is divided into three lobes, while the left contains only two.

Iinside each lung, the bronchi divide another 20 times into ever smaller branches called bronchioles, which look like twigs. This network, which consists of about 1,500 miles of air passages, leads to the alveoli, clusters of microscopic sacs that resemble fruit dangling from the tree's branches. Alveoli are the ultimate destination for inbound air; it's where individual oxygen molecules are absorbed directly into the bloodstream, while carbon dioxide is expelled from the blood and returned to the lungs to be exhaled.

Our lungs contain more than 300 million alveoli; their total surface area is roughly the size of a tennis court. Alveoli are microscopic balloons and would naturally collapse without air if not for an ingenious bit of chemistry: cells within each sac produce a surfactant that reduces the surface tension of the mucous and fluid lining the chamber, preventing a collapse. Alveoli also function as part of the immune system: each chamber houses a group of large, white blood cells called macrophages. They search for particulate matter, such as dust, that eluded filtration by the cilia and also for bacteria or harmful chemicals, all of which they engulf and destroy, protecting the body.

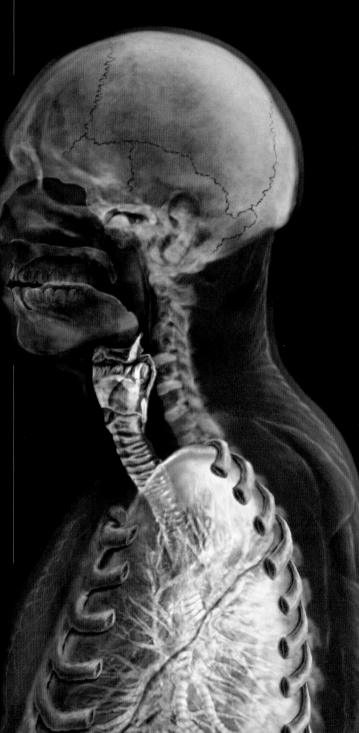

Inverted tree *If we view the respiratory system as an upside-down tree, the trachea, or windpipe, that leads from the pharynx to the lungs makes up the trunk. Because it takes in elements from the outside world, the respiratory system boasts an elaborate series of protective devices to detect, filter and destroy particles or bacteria that might irritate or infect us*

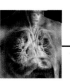

Respiratory System
Terms to Know

Adenovirus One of a group of viruses causing upper respiratory disease, including common colds.

Allergen A substance such as pollen, capable of inducing allergy or other specific sensitivity of the immune system.

Alveoli The tiny, saclike structures at the edge of the lungs where gas is exchanged with the bloodstream.

Bronchi Large airways that connect the windpipe to the lungs.

Bronchoscope A device to observe the inside of the windpipe, the bronchi and the lungs using a lighted tube inserted through the patient's nose or mouth

Dyspnea Shortness of breath.

Larynx Also called the voice box, since it contains the vocal cords; part of the breathing system in the throat.

Pharynx Passageway for air to move from mouth and nostrils to trachea (and food from the mouth to esophagus).

Pleura The thin lining that covers the lungs and the inside of the chest wall, forming a cushion for the lungs.

Pulmonologist A doctor who specializes in studying and treating diseases of the lungs.

Sleep Apnea A common respiratory disorder characterized by a periodic stop in breathing during sleep; often accompanied by loud snoring.

Trachea The airway connecting the larynx to the lungs; windpipe.

Tracheotomy A surgical procedure to open a direct airway via an incision into the trachea when air passage is blocked.

Ventilator A device that provides mechanically assisted breathing.

Sources: American Lung Association; Centers for Disease Control and Prevention

Common Respiratory Diseases and Disorders

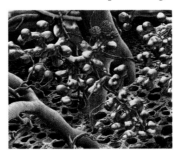

Alveoli *The small air sacs take in oxygen from blood capillaries*

Asthma Chronic inflammation and narrowing of the airways, causing a reduction in the amount of air flow.

■ **Symptoms** *Wheezing, coughing, chest tightening and shortness of breath; intercostal contractions (skin pulling between the ribs during breathing).*

■ **Treatment** Medications such as steroids and bronchodilators, which can either aim to prevent attacks or provide relief during attacks.

Emphysema Condition in which damaged lung alveoli are unable to fill with fresh air, often as a result of smoking.

■ **Symptoms** *Shortness of breath, chronic cough (often with sputum production), wheezing, decreased ability to exercise. In some cases, may be accompanied by fatigue; swelling of the ankles, feet and legs; and unintentional weight loss.*

■ **Treatment** Smoking cessation, medications to improve breathing, antibiotics to control infection, oxygen ventilation. In severe cases, lung transplantation or lung reduction surgery.

Pneumonia Infection and/or inflammation of the lungs, in which the alveoli fill with pus or other liquid, preventing oxygen from reaching the bloodstream. Usually caused by bacteria, viruses or fungi.

■ **Symptoms** *Cough with greenish or yellow mucus; fever with shaking chills; sharp or stabbing chest pain worsened during deep breathing or coughing; rapid, shallow breathing.*

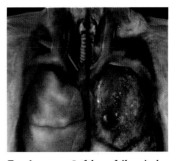

Emphysema *Left lung failure is due to chronic obstruction of air flow*

■ **Treatment** For bacterial pneumonia, antibiotics. For viral pneumonia, antiviral medications. In most all cases, drinking more fluids, bed rest and fever control.

Tuberculosis A bacterial infection that usually attacks the lungs but can also damage other body parts; spreads through the air when a person with TB of the lungs or throat coughs, sneezes or talks.

■ **Symptoms** *Usually without symptoms in initial stage. Later stages marked by severe cough lasting three weeks or longer; coughing up blood or mucus; weight loss, weakness or fatigue; fever, chills and night sweats.*

■ **Treatment** Six months or more of multiple drugs; hospitalization in severe cases or to prevent spread of the infectious disease.

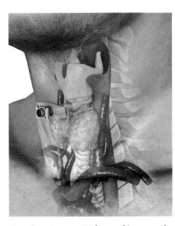

Tracheotomy *A channel is opened into the windpipe to allow breathing*

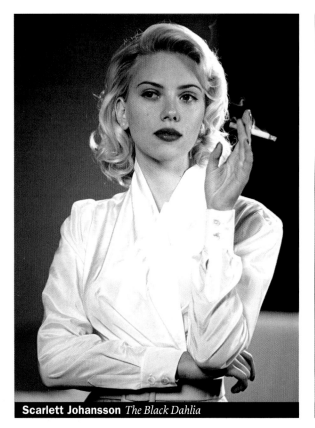

Scarlett Johansson *The Black Dahlia*

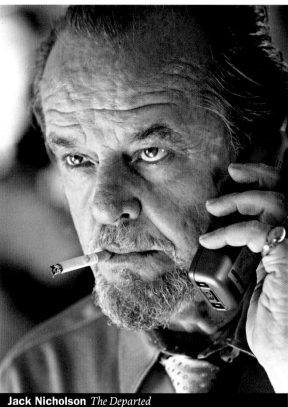

Jack Nicholson *The Departed*

■ **Briefing** Hollywood and smoking

American movies have long glamorized smoking, but today cigarettes are more common onscreen than at any other time since midcentury: 75% of all Hollywood films show tobacco use, according to a 2006 survey by the University of California, San Francisco. Audiences, especially kids, are taking notice. Two recent studies, published in the *Lancet* and *Pediatrics,* have found that among children as young as 10, those exposed to the most scenes of screen smoking are as much as 2.7 times as likely as others to pick up the habit. Worse, it's the ones from nonsmoking homes who are hit the hardest, perhaps because they are spared the dirty ashtrays and musty drapes that make real-world smoking a lot less appealing than the cinematic version.

Now the Harvard School of Public Health (HSPH), the folks behind the U.S. designated-driver campaign, are pushing to get smokers off the screen. But you can't influence behavior by telling people what to do: you do it by exposing them to enough cases of people behaving well that it creates a new norm. The designated-driver concept caught on in the 1980s because Harvard

researchers persuaded TV networks to slip the idea into their shows. That's why a designated-driver poster appeared in the bar on the long-running sitcom *Cheers.* "The idea appeared in 160 prime-time episodes over four years," says Jay Winsten, HSPH's associate dean. "Drunk-driving fatalities fell 25% over the next three years."

Harvard has long believed that getting cigarettes out of movies could have as powerful an effect on the public's behavior, but it hasn't been easy. Cigarette makers have a history of striking product-placement deals with Hollywood, and while the 1998 tobacco settlement prevents that, nothing stops directors from incorporating smoking into scenes on their own.

Now the pressure is growing. As Harvard closes in from one side, a dozen health groups, including the American Medical Association, are calling for the reduction of smoking scenes in movies and on TV, and 41 state attorneys general have signed a letter seeking public-service ads at the beginning of any DVD that includes smoking. Like smokers, studios may conclude that quitting the habit is not just a lot healthier but also a lot smarter.

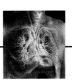

■ On the Horizon Briefs

Cold Comfort
Should toddlers be taking cold medications?

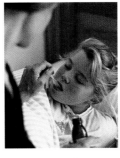

It's a bitter pill for some parents to swallow: over-the-counter cold medicines for children under 6 are likely to do more harm than good. That's the word from an FDA advisory panel, which recommended in 2007 that pediatric cold and cough products not be used for the 5-and-under age group, citing doubts about the medications' effectiveness and safety.

Reason: there is no evidence that kids' cold syrups and tablets treat symptoms. And accidental overdosing, which can occur when more than one medication is used, is too easy. While the panel voted 21 to 1 for avoiding such products for children under 2, the vote was closer for children ages 2 to 5. There's no a guarantee that the FDA will follow the panel's recommendation. In the meantime, there's always chicken soup.

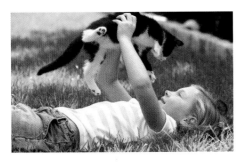

Sneezes and Wheezes A pair of common respiratory ailments may be related

Allergies and asthma may be closer kin than we knew. More than half the 20 million asthma cases in the U.S. can be attributed to common allergens such as dust mites, according to a 2007 study published in the *Journal of Allergy and Clinical Immunology*. Exposure to some of these respiratory irritants—like cat dander—at a young age may offer some protection, researchers suggested, lending support to the idea that we may be getting too clean for our own good.

Another study found that children with allergies living in affluent countries, where exposure to allergens is quite low, are almost twice as likely to develop asthma as similar children living in less-developed nations.

Unsweet Dreams Troubles with sleeping are indicators for stroke

Excessive daytime drowsiness in older adults may predict a significantly increased risk of stroke. Most people have, from time to time, unintentionally dozed off on the couch watching TV or reading a book. But persistent drowsiness during the day usually signals a chronic sleep deficit—and bigger problems. The new study found that people who suffered from "significant dozing" (those who almost always fell asleep involuntarily during the day) were 4.5 times more likely to have a stroke than people in the "no dozing" group.

Even more telling, the sleepier the person, the higher the risk of stroke. People in the "some dozing" group, who sometimes but not always fell asleep while watching TV or

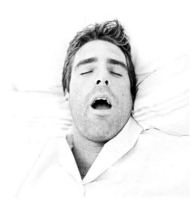

while sitting quietly after lunch, had a 2.6 times higher risk of stroke than their more alert peers. The data showed not only an increase in stroke risk with excessive daytime sleepiness but also an increased risk of heart attack and vascular death.

Past studies have examined the link between sleep and stroke, but that research has focused mainly on people with sleep apnea, a disorder that causes interruptions in breathing or shallow breaths during sleep. In one study involving patients with severe sleep apnea (five or more episodes per hour), sufferers experienced a twofold increased risk of a stroke. The strongest evidence suggests sleepiness can lead to stroke via sleep apnea, which is known to cause severe blood-pressure variations. But a growing body of research suggests that sleep disorders may also be linked to a variety of conditions, such as obesity, diabetes and hypertension, that may also contribute to vascular risk.

There's more: a 2006 study suggested a causal relationship between the severity of a sleep disorder and the odds of suffering from clinical depression. Sleep disturbances are a well-known symptom of depression, but the new study suggests that sleeping woes may contribute to depression. The bottom line: snoring and other sleep-related breathing issues should be treated seriously, both for the trouble they cause in their own right and for the deeper problems they could trigger.

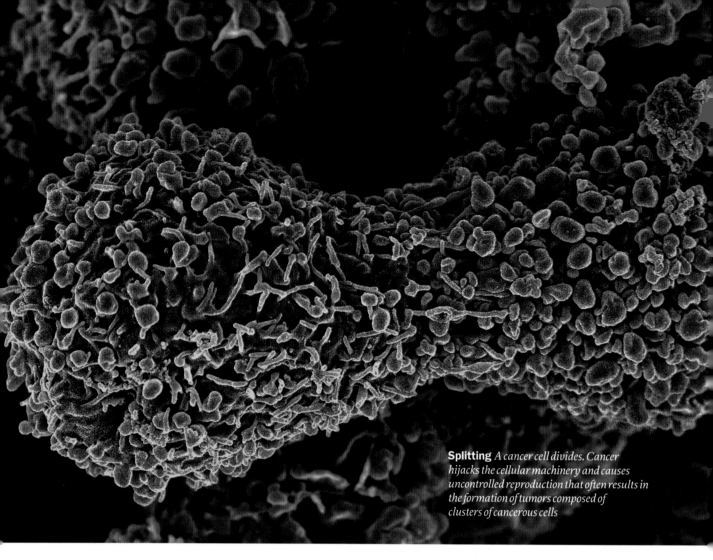

Splitting *A cancer cell divides. Cancer hijacks the cellular machinery and causes uncontrolled reproduction that often results in the formation of tumors composed of clusters of cancerous cells*

■ **Briefing** Cancer

If infectious diseases defined the medical landscape of the 1800s, then cancer has certainly taken over the mantle in the 20th and 21st centuries. Throughout much of that time, cancer rates climbed, as doctors failed to find effective ways to stop the body's cells from dividing uncontrollably. But the most recent numbers are more encouraging; the National Institutes of Health (NIH) reports that U.S. cancer rates decreased on average 2.1% per year from 2002 through 2004, nearly twice the annual decrease of 1.1% per year from 1993 through 2002. Even so, the NIH expected some 1,437,180 new cases of cancer to be diagnosed in 2008—not counting the disease's usually milder form, melanoma—causing 565,650 deaths.

As a result, the treatment of what used to be dismissed as terminal cancer has shifted from a win-or-lose battle against acute illness to something more akin to managing a chronic disease.

The change reflects a series of hard-won improvements in treatment, particularly for breast, colon, prostate and even lung cancer. The gains include an explosion of new drugs that target tumors more effectively and are less toxic than old-school chemo-therapeutic agents. Some of the new medications target communication signals within malignant cells, some cut off supply lines by interfering with the growth of blood vessels around a tumor, while others block the chemical agents that enable tumors to expand into new territory.

In addition, doctors are beginning to use new tests to match drugs more precisely to the genetic and molecular features of an individual tumor. And they are also making advances in managing the side effects of treatment, which were once as debilitating as cancer itself.

The payoff is already being seen in longer and better-quality survival. According to the American Cancer Society, the percentage of people living five years after a diagnosis of any type of cancer barely budged from 50% in the mid-1970s to 52% in the mid-'80s, but it shot to 66% for patients with a diagnosis after 1995 and is continuing to rise. For breast-cancer patients the five-year-survival numbers were even more impressive, surging from 75% in the '70s to nearly 90% by 2002.

Receiving a diagnosis of cancer is always a terrible blow. But experts on the disease maintain there is no better time than today to be living with cancer.

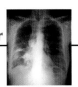

Young Survivors More kids are beating cancer, thanks to new treatments

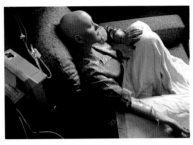

Today, 1 in 1,000 young adults in the U.S. is a childhood-cancer survivor. Since the 1970s, the chance that a child would live for five years after a diagnosis of leukemia or lymphoma has risen steadily, from an average of 25% to more than 80% today, outpacing recovery rates for most adult cancers. Most of the gains have come from wiser use of existing chemotherapy drugs in innovative combinations. Simply increasing the dose of certain agents, for instance, gives kids an advantage over some rapidly growing cancers. And while such treatments might seem excessive for still-growing bodies, doctors are convinced that young hearts, lungs and kidneys can be bombarded with higher doses of toxic drugs than most adults can tolerate. It also helps that better medications for handling the side effects and consequences of chemotherapy and radiation can help kids respond better to intensive treatment.

Tell-tale heart A simple blood test can help cancer treatment

With a disease as complex as cancer, it's easy to forget that sometimes the most effective defense can be the simplest—as when researchers in 2007 reported that the best way to figure out how a cancer is progressing is to draw a little blood. New tests can detect proteins on cancer cells released by a tumor that is just dozens of cells large. The tests not only isolate the cancerous cells but also identify their characteristics, helping doctors craft more personalized therapies that match the right treatments to the right patients at the right time, improving effectiveness, avoiding the costs of hit-or-miss treatments and reducing toxic side effects. The test's biggest appeal is its ease and simplicity: it eliminates taking samples of cancerous tissue, which can spread the disease.

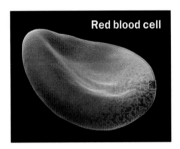

Red blood cell

A Melanoma Primer

Melanoma, skin cancer, afflicts more than 60,000 Americans each year, but it can be cured if it is caught and treated in its earliest stages. Treatment involves the removal of the tumor and a surrounding margin of skin tissue. Each stage in the growth of the cancer can be subdivided further in terms of the depth and condition of the lesion and whether other tissues have been affected

Skin

Skin

Skin

Epidermis

Tumor

Tumor

Tumor

Dermis

Cancer cells

Lymph nodes

STAGE 1	STAGE 2	STAGE 3	STAGE 4
Least severe			Most severe
The tumor begins as a lesion, often irregular in shape and color. It is usually more than 5 mm (0.2 in.) in diameter but less than 1 mm (0.04 in.) thick and affects the outer layer of the skin	The tumor penetrates the inner layer of the skin and may appear ulcerated but has not spread into other tissue. At 2-4 mm (0.08-0.16 in.) thick, the cancer can still be surgically removed	The tumor extends deeper into the skin and spreads to nearby lymph nodes. Treatment involves removal of the lesion as well as the lymph nodes. Immuno-therapy is often prescribed	The cancer spreads to distant lymph nodes and other organs, such as the liver, brain and bones. Chemotherapy and radiation may provide relief from symptoms but offer little hope for recovery

SURVIVAL RATES, *by stage*

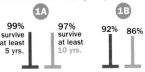

1A 99% survive at least 5 yrs.

1B 97% survive at least 10 yrs.

92% 86%

2A 78% 66%

2B 68% 59%

2C 56% 48%

3A n.a.

3B 50%-68% 44%-60%

3C 27%-52% 22%-37%

4 18% 14%

Sources: American Cancer Society; *cancerconsultants.com*

■ **Briefing** Breast Cancer

Breast cancer is the most lethal form of cancer for women in the world. An estimated 1 million cases are identified each year, and about 500,000 new and existing patients die from the disease. Some of this bad news is the result of very good news: thanks to modern medical advances and sanitation, more women are simply living long enough to reach the age at which they're most susceptible to breast cancer.

While it remains a complex disease, with many genetic and environmental causes, researchers are starting to decode some of the more obvious genetic links that are responsible for some 10% of U.S. breast-cancer cases. New screening and diagnostic devices are helping identify those at risk earlier, while new treatments are making it possible for those who contract the disease to survive it.

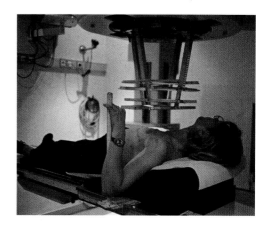

History Lessons Genes, Age and Family Can Be Risk Factors

Simply living longer is one of the strongest contributors to breast-cancer risk, since age brings greater exposure to cancer-causing agents and allows the genetic changes that precede some cancers more time to develop. One major contributor to some breast cancers is the female hormone estrogen, which can prompt breast tissue to grow abnormally after waxing and waning over a lifetime of menstrual cycles. But exactly

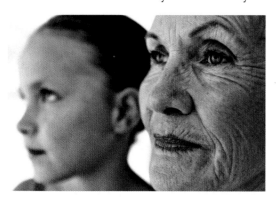

how breast cells react to the hormone is influenced by our genes. Two known genetic mutations, BRCA1 and BRCA2, have been identified, but other, still unknown genes almost certainly contribute to risk for the disease. The often cited risk factors at right are familiar to most people; some of them may be more fiction than fact.

Risk Factors

Age The older a woman is, the greater her lifetime exposure to potential carcinogens and cancer-promoting estrogen.

Genetics About 10% of breast-cancer patients in the U.S. are due to inherited mutations in the BRCA 1 or BRCA 2 genes.

Family Ties Having two or more first-degree relatives with breast cancer could hint at unknown genetic contributors to the disease.

Delayed Childbirth Putting off pregnancy increases exposure to estrogen by adding to the number of lifetime menses.

Tenuous Links

Antiperspirants Fears that blocked sweat glands cause tumors in the lymph nodes linked to the breast are unfounded.

Birth Control Oral contraceptives contain estrogen, but studies of any link to breast cancer are inconclusive.

Smoking Lighting up has not yet been found to increase breast-cancer risk, but tobacco is a known carcinogen.

Implants Studies suggest that implants, not made of living tissue, do not increase risk.

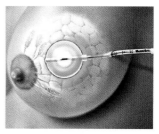

New Weapons Targeting breast tumors with seeds

The goal of any cancer treatment is to clear away malignant cells while leaving the remaining, healthy cellular landscape as intact as possible. MammoSite, a five-day, seed-based therapy, directs radiation at only cancer-rich regions of the breast. After surgically removing cancerous growth, doctors insert a balloon with a catheter into the cavity left behind by the tumor. They can then thread radioactive seeds into the balloon to zap any remaining cancer cells. After five years, treated women showed no recurrent growths in their breasts, compared to those untreated.

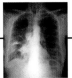

DNA Fingerprints New tests help match treatments to patients

The ability to genotype, or determine the DNA fingerprint of a tumor, is transforming the way doctors treat breast cancer. By comparing the genetic profiles of different tumors with those of normal breast tissue, researchers can pick out which genes trigger the disease and even which ones make a tumor more responsive to chemotherapy.

Doctors are currently using the three tests at right to match their patients to the most effective treatments, but in coming years genotyping may even help them identify particularly aggressive tumors.

Oncotype DX

This genetic screen analyzes 21 genes critical to breast-cell growth but relies on live rather than frozen tissue. The result consists of a recurrence score, from 0 to 100, that indicates a woman's risk of seeing her cancer return within 10 years of her diagnosis. High scores have now also been correlated with better responses to chemotherapy.

Who Benefits Women with cancer that contain estrogen-receptors and are in the earliest stage of the disease.

Mammaprint

Similar to Oncotype DX, this test scans 70 genes expressed in breast tissue. A high score means a woman has a 25% chance of seeing her cancer spread to other tissues in five years, while a low risk score indicates a 90% chance that her cancer will not spread. One disadvantage of the screen: it requires frozen-tissue samples, which most U.S. hospitals don't routinely collect following cancer surgeries.

Availability Approved for use in the U.S.

Amplichip

This test extracts DNA from a blood sample to detect an enzyme that controls the way a cancer drug, tamoxifen, is broken down. Certain genetic mutations can virtually shut down a cell's ability to metabolize tamoxifen, reducing the estrogen-based drug's success in containing tumor-cell growth. Screening women for this enzyme is sparing low responders the expense and time that would be lost on useless treatments.

Just for me Such tests are a first step toward personalized medicine.

Detection Options: MRI vs. Mammogram

Ever since the 1980s, the mammogram has been the gold standard for detecting breast tumors. Using low-dose X rays, these scans can find up to 90% of breast cancers in women who have no symptoms of the disease, giving them a critical head start in launching potentially lifesaving measures, such as surgery to remove suspicious growths. That's why the American Cancer Society (ACS) recommends that all women over 40 receive annual mammogram screenings. Mammograms can come in the form of traditional film or digital scans. The latter give doctors more opportunity to enhance and manipulate the resulting image, yet studies show that the two methods are equivalent when it comes to detecting tumors. But women at higher risk of the disease—those who already have cancer in one breast, for example, or have a family history of the disease—may benefit from another level of screening. For them, the ACS has recommended adding a magnetic resonance image (MRI) to the annual mammogram. An MRI can produce a more detailed picture of breast tissue and hence improve the chances that the smallest lesions—sometimes missed by mammography X rays—will be detected.

MRI

What It Is The use of magnetic fields to create detailed images of body tissue and changes in blood flow.

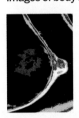

Fact Though they can be beneficial in picking up tumors in women at high risk, MRIs are not recommended as a routine screen for the general population because they are expensive and tend to produce more false positives than mammograms

Fact In the U.S. alone, about 1.4 million women at high risk of breast cancer could benefit from the additional screening.

Fact Insurers do not always cover the cost of such supplemental MRI scans.

Cost $1,000 or more.

Mammogram

What It Is An X ray–based image that has been proved to detect a majority of breast cancers.

Fact About 5% to 10% of screens performed in the U.S. each year show abnormal results; most are false positives because of factors such as breast density and improper breast positioning during the test.

Fact Mammograms account for up to 65% of the decline in U.S. deaths from breast cancer between 1975 and 2000. U.S. screening rates began dropping in 2005 because of an increase in those not insured.

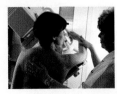

Cost $50 to $150.

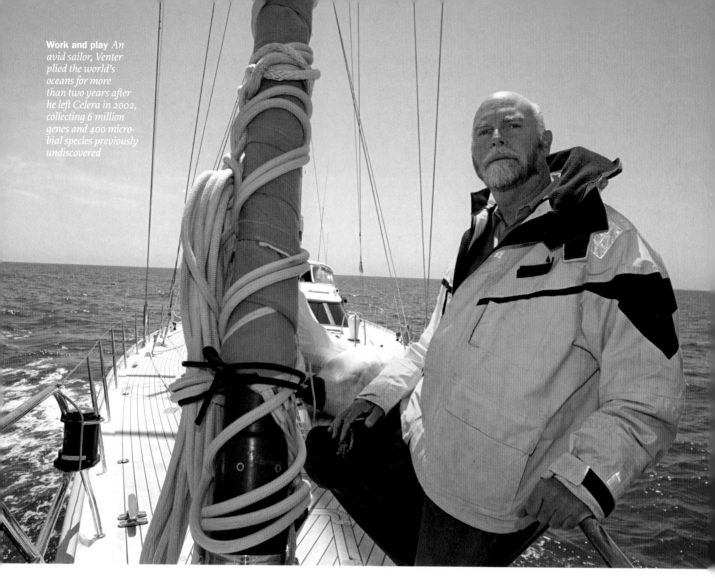

Man Makes Life*

*Well, almost. How J. Craig Venter built a genome in the lab

IF YOU WERE SETTING OUT TO DESIGN A HUMAN BEING from scratch, odds are you wouldn't take J. Craig Venter as your template. You wouldn't choose to put him at risk for Alzheimer's disease, for example, but Venter has a predisposition that places him in danger of it. You might choose his startling blue eyes, both for their color and the hard clarity of their gaze. You'd surely go for his first-rate brain, though you might pass on what his detractors consider the vainglorious temperament that comes bundled with it.

It's something of an irony then that such an imperfect organism as Venter has devoted much of his career to understanding the engineering of other organisms. He was the leader of one of two teams that in 2000 sequenced the human genome—the entire 25,000-gene cookbook that makes us people in the first place and not chimps or birds or banana trees—and he has conducted the same work with many other organisms. But Venter, 61 in 2008,

may now have done something that is at once more thrilling and promising and unsettling than all that. In a January 2008 paper in the journal *Science,* he wrote that he had gone beyond merely sequencing a genome and had designed and built one. In short, he may have created life.

Certainly, defining what we mean when we say life has become a moving target over the years. Are we alive? Yes. Is a virus alive? Maybe. Still, a half-century after the discovery of the double helix, nobody doubts that it is our DNA that determines what we are—in the same way that lines of code determine software or the digital etchings on a CD determine the music you hear. Etch new signals, and you write a new song. That, in genetic terms, is what Venter has done. Working with only the four basic nucleotides that make up all DNA—adenine, cytosine, guanine and thymine—he has assembled an entirely new chromosome for an entirely new one-celled creature. Insert that genome into a cell—like inserting a disc into a computer—and a new species of living thing will be booted up. Venter hasn't done that yet, which is why even he won't say that he has technically invented life. Yet he has already shown that a genome transplanted from an existing cell to another will shut down the host's genetic programming and bring its own online. If that cellular body-snatching works with an ordinary chromosome, it should work with a manufactured one.

The genome in Venter's lab in Rockville, Md., could revolutionize genetics, introducing a new world order in which the alchemy of life is broken down into the ultimate engineering project. Man-made genomes could lead to new species that churn out drugs to treat disease, finely tuned vaccines that target just the right lethal bug, even cells that convert sunlight into a biofuel.

Creating such small, single-purpose organisms is nowhere near as complex as creating larger, multicelled creatures: things with mobility, behavior, a purpose, a face. Those possibilities may prove too challenging and disturbing for society to allow. What Venter appears to have done, however, is crack the manufacturing code. Once you've done that, there may be little limit on what you can eventually build.

And Venter has never cared much for limits. A restless, under-achieving student during his childhood in California, he served in Vietnam as a hospital corpsman in the Navy and returned to the U.S. determined to practice medicine. Instead, in medical school he became enthralled by biochemistry and ended up taking a job with the National Institutes of Health (NIH) in Washington.

Ambitious and freethinking, Venter detested the bureaucratic maze and longed for the opportunity to test his innovative ideas for transforming the emerging field of genetics. In 1992 he secured private funding and created his own company in Rockville, the Institute for Genomic Research. Within three years he completed the first-ever genome sequencing of an entire organism—*Haemophilus influenzae*, the bacterium that causes meningitis. The firm soon became a go-to place for sequencing projects, and it wasn't long before Venter hungered for the biggest prize in biology: the map of the human genome. It was a project of mind-numbing complexity that involved determining the placement and makeup of every one of the human genome's genes, some of which can contain thousands of nucleotides.

By now, however, Venter had brainstormed a way to automate the process, pulling in supercomputers to do the work of recording each letter in all the necessary snippets of DNA and then knitting the fragments together in a simple and predictable way. In 1998 he brashly predicted that using his method, which he called shotgun sequencing, he could finish the map faster and less expensively than a competing group, the government's $3 billion sequencing effort, led by Dr. Francis Collins.

To acquire more resources, Venter joined hands with global technology giant Perkin-Elmer, forming a new company called Celera, which took its name from the middle of the word *accelerate*. The Celera-backed Venter and the NIH-backed Collins briefly explored collaborating, but those efforts fell through, and over the next two years the two camps worked feverishly, vocally at odds over whose method was better or whose intentions were purer. Collins sniffed at Venter's plans to create a genome database whose basic map he would make available for free—as the NIH planned—but to charge anyone who wanted the data processed or analyzed. In 2000, Venter finished just ahead of Collins, but a government official who knew both men brokered a truce between the groups, and they shared a joint announcement of their achievement at the White House.

The high times didn't last. In 2002, after too many tangles with the Celera board, Venter was fired, and the sailboat enthusiast followed his lifelong dream, sailing the globe to collect genetic samples from the oceans. As he shuttled between his ship and his lab, Venter was overseeing another, equally grand and potentially revolu-

Man-made genomes could lead to new species that churn out drugs, even cells that convert sunlight into a biofuel

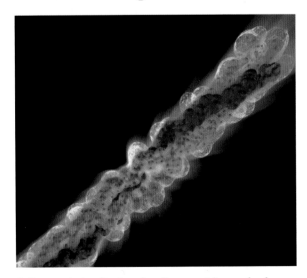

Collagen *A visualization of a collagen protein, a molecular chain of chemical building blocks that is a basic ingredient of human life*

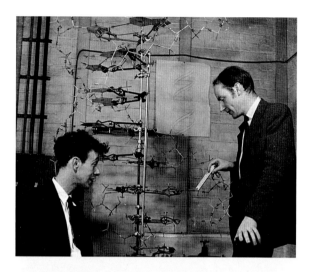

Breakthrough Deciphering the physiology of heredity

The modern era in genetics began in 1953, when Briton Francis Crick, right, and American James Watson, left, first decoded the double-helix structure of DNA. Above, the two pose with a model of the molecule. The achievement, now recognized as one of the most significant in the history of science, opened the doors to a brave new world of biology, one that has brought powerful new healing weapons to fight disease but has also evoked frightening visions of cloned humans and designer babies. Crick died in 2004; Watson turned 80 in 2008.

tionary science project: creating life. Among the organisms he and his team sequenced in the years leading up to the human-genome work was *Mycoplasma genitalium*, an unlovely bacterium whose preferred target on the animals it infects is evident by its name. That organism's genome, which the team sequenced in 1995, has one of the smallest known chromosomes of any self-replicating life-form: just 485 genes. What, Venter wondered back then, was the minimum genome an organism needed to survive and reproduce? If you could figure that out, you could determine the basic DNA chassis of all living things and then use it to design your own souped-up or dressed-down versions of life.

By 2002, advances in both genetic understanding and gene-handling technology had leaped forward. Instead of having to deconstruct *Mycoplasma genitalium*, Venter's team could build it from scratch. Whereas once they had to reverse-engineer the organism and see when it quit working, they could take the more elegant approach of assembling it from off-the-shelf nucleotides and seeing

when it switched on—thus essentially building life.

Venter decided to start small, with one or two genes, and work his way up by splicing together longer and longer pieces of DNA. That very act of sticking them together proved to be a challenge, since the strands often fall apart. The answer was to design a section of Velcro-like DNA at the ends of each fragment. Since adenine sticks only to thymine and cytosine only to guanine, all the team had to do was end each strand with a nucleotide that would adhere to the one that began the next.

Such painstaking cutting and pasting eventually did the job. Not only did Venter's team members succeed in building their own *Mycoplasma*, they also took the opportunity to rewrite its genetic score. First, they introduced a mutation that would prevent it from causing disease. Then they branded it with watermarks that would distinguish it as a product of their lab, using a code built around selected genes to spell out the names of Venter and his key colleagues. The next step will be to insert the gene into a cell and see if it indeed stirs to life.

Venter's team branded the new genome with watermarks, etching their names in genetic code on the new life form

Not everyone believes Venter will succeed—or if he does, that it will matter much. Corporate giants like DuPont are already putting synthetic biology to industrial use. In the company's Loudon, Tenn., plant, for example, billions of *E. coli* bacteria stew inside massive tanks. The bacteria's genomes contain 23 alterations that instruct it to digest sugar from corn and produce propanediol, a polyester used in plastics. The hard-working bugs churn out 100 million lbs. (45 million kg) of the stuff each year, and all it took was a little tinkering with their genomes, not the building of a new one.

Venter agrees that this all makes sense—but only if you accept a limited view of the science. He is not alone. "We are starting to turn the corner," says Jay Keasling, a bioengineer at the University of California, Berkeley. "The technologies are starting to be put in place, and it's crazy to keep doing biology the way we are doing it."

Still, after spending his career trying to digitize, quantify and standardize biology, even Venter recognizes that there may be some aspects of life that simply can't be understood without a nod to what he calls the "mystery and majesty" of the cell. Well before he became involved constructing artificial life, he christened his sailboat with a name that may reveal as much about that awareness as about his top-lofty goals: he called it *Sorcerer*. ■

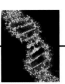

Creating a Genome from Scratch

Genes are relatively easy to make in the lab, but stringing together hundreds of them into a complete genome is a lot trickier

Mycoplasma genitalium

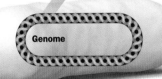

Genome

1 Venter's group started with *M. genitalium,* a bacterium with the smallest genome of any living thing

2 Venter and his team sequenced the bacterium's entire genome—which contains 582,970 chemical "letters"—on a computer

3 Next, they split the genome into 101 small fragments, and working with manufactured strips of DNA, they began assembling them. The team added short sequences of DNA at the ends of each piece to act adhesively and hold the strands together

Synthetic DNA building blocks

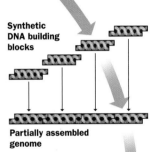

Partially assembled genome

6 The complete genome was extracted and sequenced again as a quality-control step

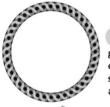

4 Smaller strips were linked first, making longer and longer individual strands that were themselves linked until the genome was complete. At each step, the group checked the growing genome to make sure that the order was correct

5 The final assembly of the last four pieces took place in yeast cells, which made multiple copies of the synthetic strands and brought them together

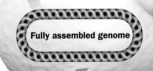

Fully assembled genome

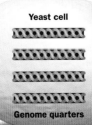

Yeast cell

Genome quarters

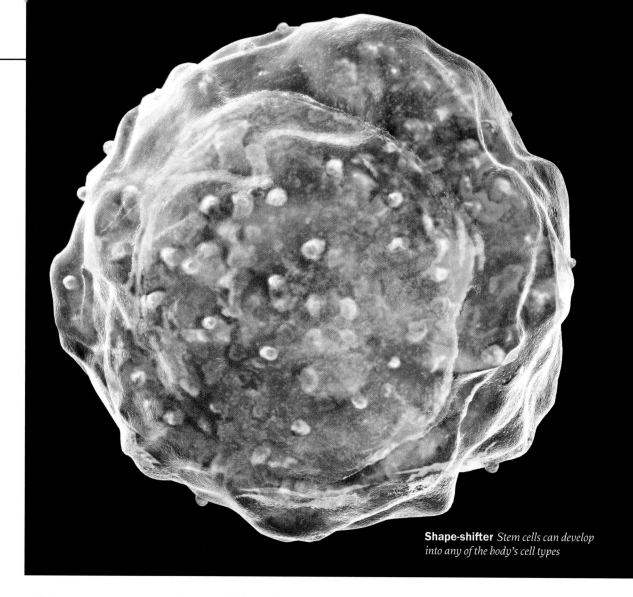

Shape-shifter *Stem cells can develop into any of the body's cell types*

Stem-Cell Breakthroughs

New discoveries sidestep using embryonic stem cells to heal

TWENTY-FIVE DAYS. THAT'S HOW LONG IT TOOK Shinya Yamanaka of Kyoto University to undo more than three decades of the exquisitely programmed biology packed into a middle-aged woman's cheek cell—and just maybe change the world. In those three weeks, Yamanaka turned back the clock on an aging cell. In the ultimate feat of reprogramming, he tricked it into acting like that wonder of cellular shape-shifting, the embryonic stem cell: capable of dividing, developing and maturing into any of the body's more than 200 different cell types.

What's remarkable is that Yamanaka wasn't the only one. On the same November day that the Japanese researcher published his milestone in the journal *Cell*, James Thomson, the pioneering molecular biologist at the University of Wisconsin who in 1998 discovered the first human embryonic stem cells, reported similar success in *Science*, reversing development in foreskin cells

from newborns. The papers were a pair of remarkable stem-cell firsts, further proof that scientists had surged ahead of ethicists and politicians in finding ever more clever ways to generate stem cells.

Also in 2007, other researchers working with mouse embryos nurtured a stem-cell line from the earliest stage of development yet: the one-celled zygote. Still another team propagated stem cells from a single cell extracted from a days-old eight-cell human embryo, leaving the embryo itself intact and developing. And Oregon scientists reported they could grow embryonic stem cells from an adult monkey, inching closer to perfecting the process with human cells.

But those three breakthroughs, newsworthy as they were, still relied on living embryos: tiny bits of inchoate life fraught with all the familiar ethical issues. Yamanaka's and Thomson's work sidestepped that altogether, raising the tantalizing question, Is the long-raging stem-

100

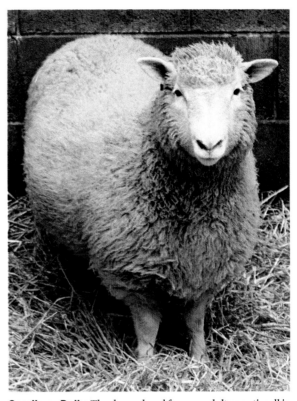

cell debate at last over? No embryos, no eggs, no hand-wringing over where the cells came from and whether it was ethical to make them in the first place? Yamanaka thought it might be. "We can now for sure begin to generate patient-specific stem cells," he said. "And we should be able to use them in cell-transplant therapy."

Stem cells generated by Yamanaka's or Thomson's method are ideal for producing transplant cells not just because they are free of political and moral baggage. Since they originate in a patient, they can also give rise to any type of body tissue and then be transplanted back into the donor with little risk of rejection. All it took, in the end, was a bit of gene-tinkering and a dousing of protein factors that together coaxed cells back to an embryonic state in which everything is biologically possible.

It wasn't always obvious that such direct reprogramming could be achieved, for it seemed to involve hundreds of protein factors and an unknown amount of gene-jiggering to recalibrate the cell properly, all of which would have to be discovered by trial and error.

Fortunately, things were easier than that. The fountain-of-youth factors both teams used are well-known genes active in early development. Both groups relied on inserting a separate set of four genes into aging cells, using the most efficient genetic bullies around: viruses, which can easily penetrate a cell's membrane and insert new genetic software into its nucleus. The technique is comparatively efficient—about one stem-cell line per 5,000 cells, in Yamanaka's case, or one stem-cell line for each cultured petri dish of cells. While that may not sound impressive, it's a sure thing compared

Goodbye, Dolly *The sheep, cloned from an adult somatic cell in 1996 at the Roslin Institute in Scotland, lived until the age of 6*

with the painstaking method that produced Dolly.

Still, that doesn't mean these cells are ready for transplant into patients. The viruses used to ferry the genes are retroviruses and lentiviruses, which can introduce genetic mutations that can cause cancer. But, said Dr. Douglas Melton, co-director of the Harvard Stem Cell Institute, "eventually we may not need to add genes or viruses at all to cells. It will be possible to find chemicals that tickle the cells to turn the right pathways on."

The fact that the two groups came up with a different set of factors makes clear that there are probably myriad ways to reprogram a cell. And sorting out those methods to determine the best ones will take time—which is why some experts believe that stem cells from embryos will remain useful for a while. Although both Yamanaka and Thomson have induced their cells to develop further—into heart and nerve cells, among others—they admit that we still know too little about how this development process works to exploit the method's full potential. "My hope is to avoid using human embryonic stem cells," says Yamanaka. "But at this point, I am not 100% sure that is possible yet." Given the speed of new discoveries in the field, however, he may not have long to wait. ■

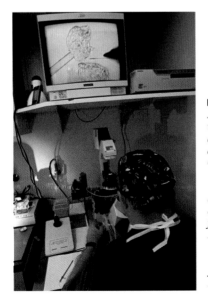

Life's instruction kit *A researcher works with stem cells from a donated human embryo in La Jolla, Calif. The work of Yamanaka and Thomson may help avoid the use of embryonic stem cells for healing. "When I started this work, I thought it would be a 20-year—not a few-year—problem," said Thomson*

■ On the Horizon Briefs

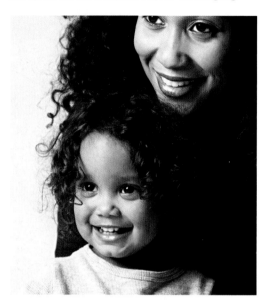

Mysterious Mitochondria The tiny organelles that power cells are suspected in a host of diseases

In recent years doctors have identified hundreds of different subtypes of mitochondrial disease, a disorder that they are only beginning to study. What they all have in common is a malfunction of the mitochondria—tiny substructures, or organelles, found inside every cell in the body that convert food into a chemical called ATP that cells use for energy. Mitochondria differ from the rest of the cell in that they possess their own DNA— inherited directly from the mother, with no input from the father—that's entirely separate from the DNA in the nucleus. When mitochondria go bad, all sorts of metabolic havoc may ensue: muscle wasting, nerve damage, seizures, stroke, blindness and more.

Officially, as many as 2 million Americans suffer from mitochondrial disease. But researchers are beginning to suspect the ailment may underlie an astonishing range of familiar illnesses: reports are now implicating the disorder as a factor in diseases such as Alzheimer's and Parkinson's. Indeed, says Harvard Medical School researcher Dr. Vamsi Mootha, "it looks like mitochondria are really important in diabetes, hypertension and many other common diseases—even in the aging process itself." Mitochondrial genetic diseases are characterized by alterations in the mitochondrial genome, which can cause premature aging, maternally inherited metabolic diseases and other serious ailments.

Screen Saver A new test helps identify birth defects early in pregnancy

Researchers continue to find better ways to test for the presence of potential birth defects in the womb, including Down syndrome, a genetic condition in which every cell in a person's body has 47 rather than 46 chromosomes. The disorder can slow both body and brain development. Beginning in 2007, the American College of Obstetricians and Gynecologists has recommended that all pregnant women get a new test, a first-trimester prenatal screening for the genetic abnormality, regardless of their age.

The new screen replaces amniocentesis, a medical procedure in which a doctor inserts a long needle through the belly and withdraws amniotic fluid, which is then evaluated for birth defects. Inserting the needle into the amniotic sac containing the growing fetus, however, carries a slight but real chance for miscarriage. The new screening, by contrast, does not require any such invasion of the fetal environment. It combines two routine blood tests and an ultrasound that measures something called nuchal translucency, a property of the fluid at the back of the baby's neck that tells doctors with better than 90% accuracy whether the baby is at increased risk of Down syndrome. If the test is positive, mothers still have to decide whether to undergo amniocentesis or another test, chorionic villus sampling, to confirm the diagnosis one way or the other. But if it is negative, no further action is needed.

All U.S. women should now have a choice between the two tests. For those who prefer the new procedure, TIME health columnist Sanjay Gupta, M.D., recommends choosing a hospital at which the technicians have been trained to perform it, a factor that can have a big effect on the trustworthiness of the results.

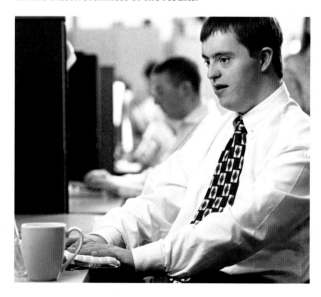

■ **Briefing** The Cell

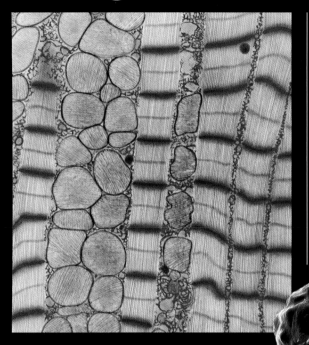

"small organs," or organelles, that perform the specialized labor of the cell. Among them are the endoplasmic reticulum, flattened tubes that manufacture, store and transport essential substances, including proteins and fats. Other organelles, such as Golgi bodies, are flattened membrane sacs that process protein and pack it into vesicles that maneuver to the plasma membrane, where they release their contents into the bloodstream.

Additional organelles include microtubules, which help support the cell and retain its shape. But perhaps the most interesting are the mitochondria, the power plants that keep the cell's various activities running smoothly. Within the mitochondria's folded inner membranes, or cristae, aerobic respiration takes place, and food is converted into energy in the form of adenosine triphosphate (ATP), which fuels the cell's activity. If this process sounds like a factory at work—well, cells are indeed the factories that keep the body running.

But in order to keep things humming along, cells must also be able to replenish themselves. Most of the body's cells reproduce by dividing, in a process called mitosis. The exception are the sex cells, sperm and egg, which divide in a different fashion, meiosis. In the process of mitosis, a cell divides to produce two identical "daughters." The process begins in the nucleus, where each of the 46 chromosomes that contain the DNA of the human genome copies itself. The process resembles the unzipping of a tightly wound zipper, which is then reassembled with a new strand of DNA forming a replica of the original. At this point, the cell is ready to divide: the nucleus leads the way, splitting into two equal segments, and the cytoplasm lingers as a single unit that morphs into a dumbbell shape before separating to form two cells.

Most cells divide about 50 times before they lose their ability to regenerate and start to die—spent, but having lived long and biologically productive lives.

Cells are the body's primal units, the micro-scopic Erector sets from which we are built. The human body contains trillions of cells, separated into specialized groups to perform tightly defined functions. Red blood cells carry the oxygen that nourishes us; skin cells, or epithelial cells, cover the outer part of the body and line the interior of the body's tubes and cavities; bone-marrow cells produce the red blood cells.

Each cell is a miniature world unto itself. Surrounding it is a skin, or plasma membrane, an oily fluid that quickly seals if it is ever broken. The control center of each cell is its nucleus, which contains the DNA, or genetic material that directs its growth. The area between the nucleus and the plasma membrane is awash in cytoplasm, a fluid containing various

Cells at work *At top, a cross-section view of heart muscle shows large oval mitochondria and bright pink muscle fiber. At right, the stages of mitosis: (1) a resting cell, (2) RNA synthesis, (3) DNA synthesis, (4) the cell divides into two parts, (5) each new cell bears all the chromosomes of the original*

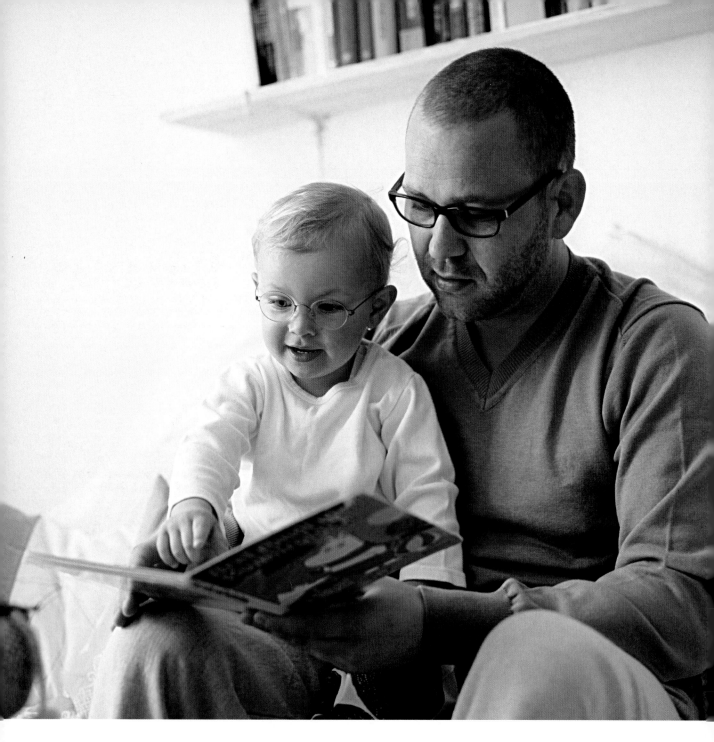

What Do Babies Know?

Less than we thought, say researchers at the new Babylab

WATCHING INFANTS PIECE LIFE TOGETHER, SEEING their senses, emotions and motor skills take shape, is a source of mystery and endless fascination—at least to parents and developmental psychologists. But how much do we really know about what's going on behind those wide, innocent eyes? How much of their understanding of and response to the world comes preloaded at birth? How much is built from scratch by experience? Such are the questions being ex-

plored at Babylab, a unit founded in 2005 at the University of Manchester in England to investigate how babies think. Though the facility is a bit of a toddler itself and has tested only 100 infants, it's already challenging current thinking on what babies know and how they come to know it.

The Swiss pioneer of such studies, Jean Piaget, started experimenting on children in the 1920s. His work led him to conclude that infants younger than 9 months have no innate knowledge of how the world works or any sense of "object permanence" (that people and things still exist when they're not seen). Instead, babies must gradually construct this knowledge from experience.

Piaget's "constructivist" theories were highly influential on postwar educators and psychologists, but over the past 20 years or so they have been largely set aside by a new generation of "nativist" psychologists and cognitive scientists whose more sophisticated experiments led them to theorize that infants arrive already equipped with some knowledge of the physical world and even rudimentary programming for math and language. Babylab director Sylvain Sirois has been putting these smart-baby theories through a rigorous set of tests. His conclusions so far tend to be more Piagetian: "Babies," he says, "know squat."

Are infants born with some knowledge of the world? Or—as one researcher argues—do babies "know squat"?

Sirois does not take issue with the way these experiments were conducted. "The methods are correct and replicable," he says. "It's the interpretation that's the problem." In a critical review published in the *European Journal of Developmental Psychology*, he and co-author Iain Jackson pour cold water over recent experiments that claim to have observed innate or precocious social cognition skills in infants.

So how do babies bridge the gap between knowing squat and drawing triangles? "Babies have to learn everything, but as Piaget was saying, they start with a few primitive reflexes that get things going," says Sirois. For example, hard-wired in the brain is an instinct that draws a baby's eyes to a human face. From brain-imaging studies we also know that the brain has some sort of visual buffer that continues to represent objects after they have been removed—a lingering perception rather than conceptual understanding. So when babies encounter novel or unexpected events, Sirois explains, "there's a mismatch between the buffer and the information they're getting at that moment. And what you do when you've got a mismatch is you try to clear the buffer. And that takes attention." So learning, says Sirois, is essentially the laborious business of resolving mismatches. "The thing is, you can do a lot of it with this wet, sticky thing called a brain. It's a fantastic, statistical-learning machine." That's a proposition that both nativists and constructivists can agree on. ∎

Tutors for Toddlers Are anxious parents pushing kids too soon?

Call it kindercramming. These days one of the fastest-growing markets for after-school tutors is preschoolers and kindergartners, whose parents are hoping that if their kids learn to read before first grade, it will ultimately help them get into college and get good jobs. After years of *Baby Einstein* marketing, some parents have become convinced that the more math and reading skills their tots master, the better. Result: franchises geared toward giving toddlers an academic edge are popping up across the country.

The toddler-tutoring frenzy was intensified by a 2007 study in *Developmental Psychology*. Researchers who examined longitudinal data on nearly 36,000 preschoolers in the U.S., Canada and Britain found that the best predictor of success in later school years wasn't the ability to pay attention in class but was in entering kindergarten with basic math and reading skills.

Experts caution, however, that these findings should not be taken as an endorsement of academic drills for preschoolers, even as kindercramming companies continue to hype the perceived need for math and reading drills for toddlers. Says the study's lead author, Greg Duncan, a social-policy expert at Northwestern University: "The kind of skills that matter in affecting later learning are things parents can pretty easily convey to their children in the home." These include such basics as the knowledge of letters and the order of numbers. That should give parents who are expecting too much too soon plenty of busywork.

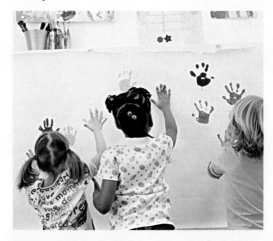

Making their mark *How soon is too soon for children to begin the serious work of math and reading drills?*

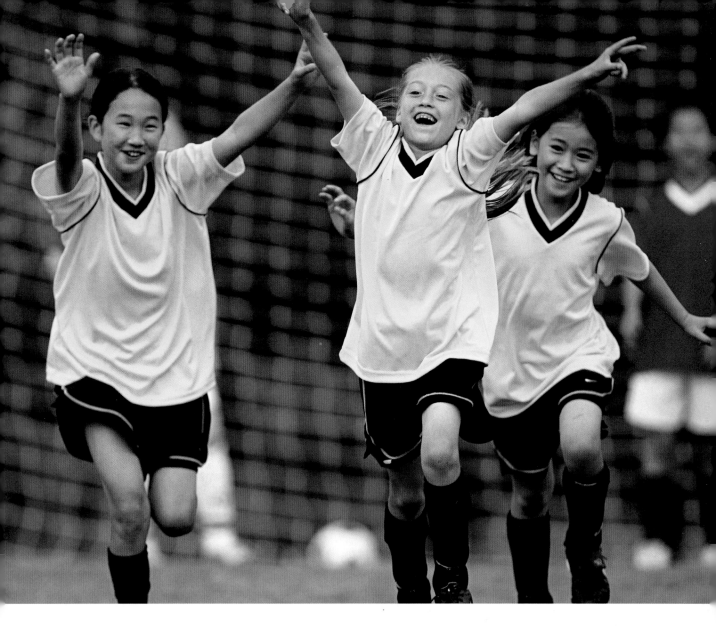

For Kids, Busy Is Better

Despite dire warnings, kids do fine when their days fill up

ONE OF THE NEUROSES THAT AFFLICT A SOCIETY obsessed with youth is the fear that childhood isn't what it used to be. Every few years a new book or magazine article warns that kids are being rushed through childhood with barely a second to skin a knee. Recent years brought several new offerings in the lost-childhood genre: a 2007 report in the journal *Pediatrics* on the decline in free playtime and two books from David Elkind, a psychologist whose *The Hurried Child* (first published in 1981) has made him the dean of too-fast-too-soon studies.

The idea that kids should slow down and trade electronic pleasures for pastoral ones is a fine example of transference. (Aren't you really the one who wants to lose the BlackBerry and go fishing?) But there's not much evidence that the ways childhood has changed in the past 25 years—less unstructured play, more gadgets, rough college admissions—are actually hurting kids. Just the opposite.

The Hurried Child has sold some 500,000 copies, and at 76, Elkind still enjoys an active speaking schedule. The book hypothesizes that nearly every social ill affecting kids—drug use, suicide, early sex, bad grades—is rooted in society's relentless message that the young should act older. But kids' lives have become even more rushed, scheduled and digitized than Elkind could have imagined more than 25 years ago, and many psychosocial metrics of childhood have actually improved.

According to the National Institutes of Health, teen pregnancy rates today are much lower than they were in the late 1970s, though they did show a slight uptick in 2007, the first in 15 years. (And that's not simply because of condoms: the overall incidence of sexual intercourse among adolescents declined significantly from 1995 to 2002, according to the Centers for Disease Control.) Teen drug use has dropped steadily over the past decade. There's less school violence and juvenile crime. And the death rate due to suicide among 15-to-19-year-olds was lower in 2003 (when 7 kids in 100,000 killed themselves) than in 1980 (when 9 in 100,000 did so). SAT scores have risen during the same period.

Elkind further indulged his atavism in his 2007 book, *The Power of Play*, a lamentation on the gradual replacement of toy trucks and dollhouses with "robopets and battery-operated cars," which "don't leave much to the imagination." (But didn't the toy truck seem outrageously modern to a Victorian who grew up playing with wood blocks and marbles?) Similarly, the American Academy of Pediatrics argued in its journal against the ebb of recess, noting that "undirected play allows children to learn how to work in groups, to share, to negotiate, to resolve conflicts ..." But most schools—at least 70%—haven't cut recess.

According to the University of Maryland's Sandra Hofferth, whose research team has studied children's time use, although noncomputer playtime has shrunk, kids now spend more hours studying, reading and participating in youth groups, art and other hobbies. Kids also take more time to shop and groom themselves but not to watch the tube: Hofferth and her colleagues have found that 9-to-12-year-olds were watching TV less than 15 hours a week in 2002—down from 20 hours in 1981.

Not all the news is good. Young people have much higher rates of sexually transmitted disease than adults. And kids spend less time outdoors these days (only 25 minutes a week for the average 6-to-12-year-old) and more time with Wiis and iPods. Kids' lives are also indisputably more scheduled now, in part because the baby boomlet has made élite college admissions tougher. But in 2006 a team led by Joseph Mahoney of the Yale psychology department wrote a paper for the journal *Social*

By almost any measure of social and psychological behavior you choose, kids' lives have improved since 1981

Policy Report showing that most of the scheduling is beneficial: kids' well-being tends to improve when they participate in extracurriculars. The paper notes that only 6% of adolescents spend more than 20 hours a week in organized activities, and these enthusiasts report better well-being and less drug use. They even eat meals with their parents more often than those who don't participate in after-school activities at all.

Childhood is an invention of modernity; for most of history, kids lived and worked alongside adults. That's not to say we shouldn't value a period of carefree shelter for our young. But the next time you're hauling the kid from basketball to SAT prep to violin class, ask yourself whether it is she who really wants a break—or you. ∎

Dance the weight away "Exergames" for kids turn out to be a fun way to rock off the pounds

Here's a counterintuitive thought: if you want your child to lose weight, turn on the video games. Several new studies show that "exergaming" systems like Dance Dance Revolution, shown at right, and the EyeToy, both of which require users to dance, kick, dodge and generally shake their booties, may help them shed unwanted pounds.

In January 2007 the Mayo Clinic, in Rochester, Minn., found that obese children burn six times as many calories playing Dance Dance Revolution as they do with a traditional video game. That's no surprise perhaps—but the secret is that, unlike phys-ed classes or visits to the gym, kids genuinely enjoy the video games.

Even more encouraging: college students burn twice as many calories using an EyeToy, a digital camera device that allows users to watch themselves interacting with video games, as they do walking on a treadmill. But how do exergames compare with an hour of basketball? The jury is still out.

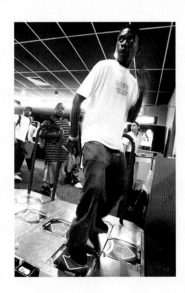

The Boys Are All Right

Critics say young men are in trouble, but new studies disagree

BOY, OH, BOY: THESE ARE TOUGH TIMES FOR BOYS, IF you heed the steady stream of books and essays filled with dire warnings about the fate of America's young men. The case against boys is disturbing and familiar: more boys than girls are in special-education classes. More boys than girls are prescribed drugs to manage their moods. More boys than girls drop out of high school. Boys don't read as well as girls. And America's prisons are packed with boys and former boys. Meanwhile, fewer boys than girls take the SAT. Fewer boys than girls apply to college. Fewer boys than girls, in annual surveys of college freshmen, express a passion for learning. And fewer boys than girls are earning college degrees.

Observers of the boy crisis contend that families, schools and popular culture are failing our boys, leaving them restless bundles of anxiety—misfits in the classroom and video-game junkies at home. They suffer from an epidemic of "anomie," as Harvard psychologist William Pollack told TIME, adrift in a world of change without the help they need to find their way. While teachers focus on test-oriented rote learning, schools are cutting science labs, physical education and recess, where the experiential learning styles of boys come into play. No wonder, the theory goes, our boys get jittery, grow disruptive and eventually tune out.

There's more to the story, however. Speaking for the defense is *America's Children: Key National Indicators of Well-Being, 2007*. The work of many federal agencies, this national report card gathers a trove of data that indicate the downward slide has leveled off—and in many cases, turned around. Boys today look pretty good compared with their dads and older cousins. By some measures, in fact, our boys are doing better than ever.

The juvenile crime rate in 2005 (the most recent year cited in the report) was down by two-thirds from its peak in 1993. Other Justice Department statistics show that the population of juvenile males in prison is only half of its historic high. The number of high school senior boys using illegal drugs has fallen by almost half compared

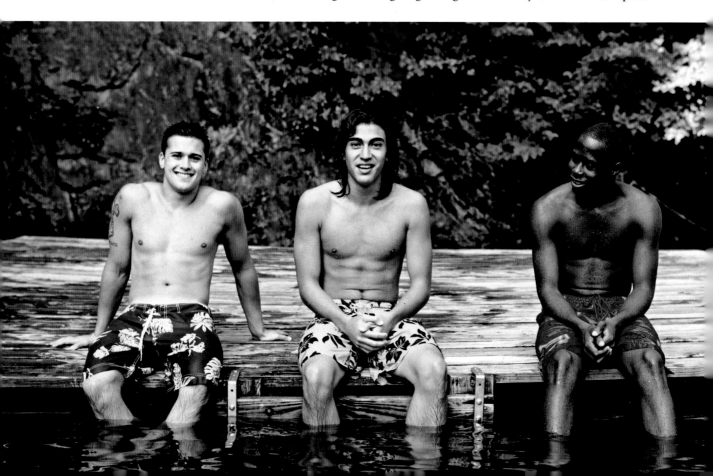

The Great Turnaround

Across dozens of educational and social measures, today's school-age boys are doing far better than in previous decades. Some examples:

Percentage of students dropping out of high school, ages 16 to 24

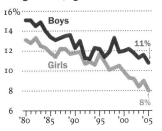

4%

Increase in boys' graduation rate since 1980

Percentage of high schoolers enrolled in college immediately after graduation

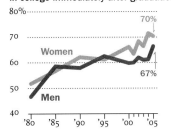

3%

Increase in boys' average SAT score since 1980

Percentage of 16-to-19-year-olds neither enrolled in school nor working

12%

Decline in percentage of boys who both work and attend school, since 1985

Percentage of 12th-graders who reported having five or more alcoholic beverages in a row in the past two weeks

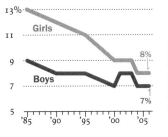

42%

Decline in illicit-drug use among boys since 1980

Percentage of high school students using birth control (among those who reported having sex in the past three months)

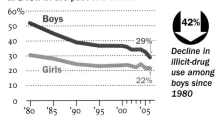

33%

Decline in teen birthrate since 1991

Sources: Federal Interagency Forum on Child and Family Statistics; National Center for Education Statistics

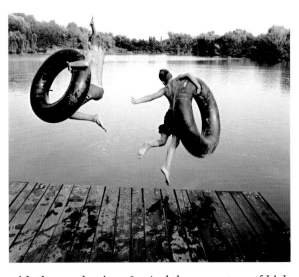

with the number in 1980. And the percentage of high school boys drinking heavily is now the lowest on record. Today's girls are also doing well by these measures; in fact, together our kids are reversing one of the direst problems of the previous generation: the teen-pregnancy epidemic. According to the new report, fewer than half of all high school boys and girls in 2005 were sexually active. For the boys, that's a decrease of 10 percentage points from the early 1990s. Boys who are having sex report that they are more responsible about it: 7 in 10 are using condoms, compared with about half in 1993. As a result, teen pregnancy and abortion rates are at their lowest recorded levels.

What about school? Boys in the fourth, eighth and 12th grades all score better—though not dramatically better—on math tests than did the comparable boys of 1990. Reading, however, is a problem. By the senior year of high school, boys have fallen nearly 20 points behind their female peers. Yet even here there may be grounds for a hopeful outlook. Boys at the fourth- and eighth-grade levels are showing modest improvement in reading and now trail their female classmates by slightly smaller margins than before. More good news: fewer boys today are deadbeats. The percentage of young men between 16 and 19 who neither work nor attend school has fallen by about a quarter since 1984, and the greatest gains in this category have been made by black youths.

Today's boys may wear their pants too damned baggy and go around with iPod buds in their ears. They know everything about Xbox 360 and nothing about paper routes. They may not slog to school through deep snow as their parents did back before the globe warmed up. But judging from the numbers, they are pulling themselves up from the handbasket to hell. ∎

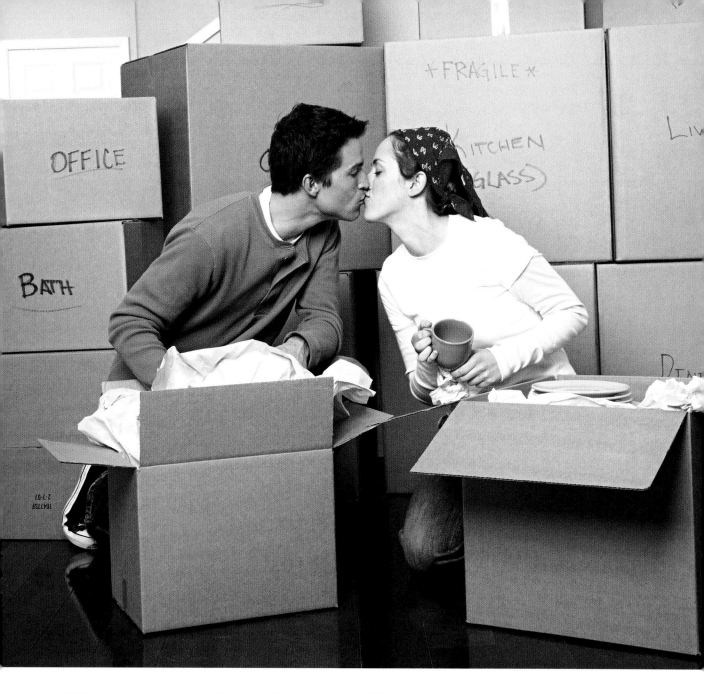

Prescription: Marry Me!

The apple of your eye may help keep the doctor away

POPULAR SENTIMENT PORTRAYS A GOOD MARRIAGE AS a source of bliss for the couple, security for the kids and stability for society. And it often is. Yet plenty of spouses—at least after the first wedded year—just come to see it as a whole lot of work. To them, marriage turns out to be a source of stress (and it is), conflict (that too) and endless crises that need to be resolved (ditto).

But marriage is also something more. Decades of data collection have shown that—for all its challenges—a good marriage is like a health-insurance policy. A 2006 paper that tracked mortality over an eight-year period found that people who never married were 58% likelier

to die during that time than married folks were. And no wonder. Marriage means no more drinking at singles' bars until closing, no more eating uncooked ramen noodles out of the bag and calling it a meal. According to a 2004 report from the Centers for Disease Control and Prevention (CDC), married people are less likely to smoke or drink heavily than people who are single, divorced or widowed. These sorts of moderating lifestyle changes are known to lower rates of cardiovascular disease, cancer and respiratory diseases. And while you might sometimes gripe that your spouse drives you nuts, just the opposite is true. Married people have lower rates of all types of mental illnesses and suicide. And none of that touches on the reduced likelihood of contracting sexually transmitted diseases that comes simply from climbing out of the dating pool.

All the health benefits of marriage are consistent across age, race, education and income groups. Some of the reasons for this are obvious: a partner can be a check on bad behavior, a proximate observer of depression and other emotional ills. But much of what makes marriage so healthy for us takes place within our own bodies, without our knowledge. A lot of those benefits come down to managing stress, which puts into motion a biological cascade involving hormones, glands and neural circuits that throws our bodies into emergency mode.

Some recent studies indicate that marriage helps the body circumvent this mess by hushing the brain's hypothalamus gland, which instructs your adrenal glands to pump out the stress hormone cortisol. "This suggests," University of Virginia neuroscientist James Coan says, "that your spouse may function as an analgesic."

All of this is especially good news for men. A study published in the January 2008 issue of the journal *Health Psychology* showed that while married men get relief from their workday barrage of stress hormones when they come home after a particularly busy day at the office, working women are able to de-stress similarly only if they describe their marriage as a happy one.

For all its benefits, marriage is not a gift certificate for good health. For one thing, it's fattening. According to a CDC study of health and marriage, married people, while least likely to be physically inactive, are most likely to be overweight or obese. Married men, in particular, seem to pack on the pounds after they say their vows: they are nearly 20% more likely to be overweight or obese than are men who have never married.

Data also show that the stress of a bad marriage can undo much of the good that comes with a happy one. In a series of studies, psychoneuroimmunologist Janice Kiecolt-Glaser and her husband, immunologist Ronald Glaser, also of the Ohio State University College of Medicine, found that "negative marital interactions," such as arguments, name-calling and nonverbal cues like eye-rolling, help increase cortisol levels and decrease immune function and even wound-healing. The effects were seen in both sexes, but were found to be stronger in women.

And when the protective bonds of marriage break, watch out. Those supposedly apocryphal tales of spouses who die within days of each other have more than a little truth to them. A 2007 British study found that at any given moment, a bereaved spouse has a greater risk of death from just about any cause (except, oddly, lung cancer) than a still married person.

Certainly not all suddenly single spouses will suffer such a fate—no more than all people who never pair off are destined for a shortened life filled with illness and stress. Humans are socially resourceful creatures who get the attention, hand-holding and even scolding they need in a lot of different ways. Still, it's hard to argue with an institution that keeps a companion and caretaker constantly nearby, even if now and again—when arguments flare over the laundry or the toothpaste or the paycheck—we may lose sight of that happy fact. ■

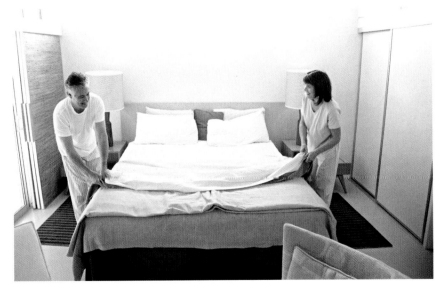

A good marriage, researchers are discovering, is like a health-insurance policy, offering a wide range of benefits

How to Look Young at Work

More boomers are working longer, and geezers just aren't cool

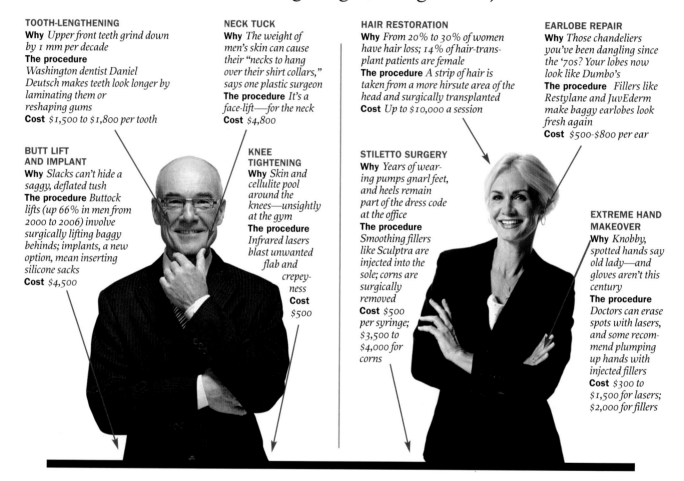

TOOTH-LENGTHENING
Why *Upper front teeth grind down by 1 mm per decade*
The procedure
Washington dentist Daniel Deutsch makes teeth look longer by laminating them or reshaping gums
Cost *$1,500 to $1,800 per tooth*

BUTT LIFT AND IMPLANT
Why *Slacks can't hide a saggy, deflated tush*
The procedure *Buttock lifts (up 66% in men from 2000 to 2006) involve surgically lifting baggy behinds; implants, a new option, mean inserting silicone sacks*
Cost *$4,500*

NECK TUCK
Why *The weight of men's skin can cause their "necks to hang over their shirt collars," says one plastic surgeon*
The procedure *It's a face-lift—for the neck*
Cost *$4,800*

KNEE TIGHTENING
Why *Skin and cellulite pool around the knees—unsightly at the gym*
The procedure *Infrared lasers blast unwanted flab and crepeyness*
Cost *$500*

HAIR RESTORATION
Why *From 20% to 30% of women have hair loss; 14% of hair-transplant patients are female*
The procedure *A strip of hair is taken from a more hirsute area of the head and surgically transplanted*
Cost *Up to $10,000 a session*

STILETTO SURGERY
Why *Years of wearing pumps gnarl feet, and heels remain part of the dress code at the office*
The procedure *Smoothing fillers like Sculptra are injected into the sole; corns are surgically removed*
Cost *$500 per syringe; $3,500 to $4,000 for corns*

EARLOBE REPAIR
Why *Those chandeliers you've been dangling since the '70s? Your lobes now look like Dumbo's*
The procedure *Fillers like Restylane and JuvEderm make baggy earlobes look fresh again*
Cost *$500-$800 per ear*

EXTREME HAND MAKEOVER
Why *Knobby, spotted hands say old lady—and gloves aren't this century*
The procedure *Doctors can erase spots with lasers, and some recommend plumping up hands with injected fillers*
Cost *$300 to $1,500 for lasers; $2,000 for fillers*

SAY WHAT YOU WANT ABOUT THE GLORIES OF GROWing old—the gaining of wisdom, the drooling grandbabies, the half-off tickets to matinees of *The Bucket List*. When it comes to the physical manifestations of advanced years, though, there ain't no euphemizing the indignities. Knees go. Teeth crumble. Ear hairs sprout. Or as Charla Krupp, author of the 2008 best seller *How Not to Look Old*, puts it, "Aging sucks."

It's worse for baby boomers, who must grow old in full view of their colleagues. AARP says 79% of boomers plan to work into the traditional retirement years—good news for employers facing a shortage of skilled workers, bad news for the condo market in Florida. "One way to stay competitive in the workplace is to look young, hip and current," says Krupp.

Job anxiety is helping drive what analysts estimate is a $50 billion antiaging industry. Boomers are already the largest consumers of hair-coloring products, cosmetic dentistry and plastic surgery. That includes the men too. The American Society of Plastic Surgeons reported that men received 1 out of 10 procedures in 2006. New York City cosmetic surgeon Dr. Neil Sadick says up to a quarter of his patients are male, many of them boomers whose goal is to look good for the office.

Good thing that new antiaging remedies never get old. The trick is not to look as though you're trying too hard. "You don't want a man coming in with a bad toupee and lots of makeup," says Lou Kacyn, a partner at global headhunters Egon Zehnder International. So save the leather pants for the weekend Harley ride. ∎

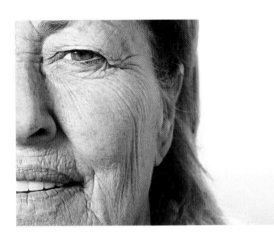

Each product has one or more active ingredients, straight from the labs of the doctors and scientists behind them, that purport to make varied and sundry improvements to the skin. In fact, many of the ingredients would qualify as prescriptions in different combinations or strengths. But because cosmeceuticals are not recognized by the Food and Drug Administration (FDA), they are not federally regulated or approved. The credibility of each product thus relies entirely on that of the scientists behind it.

Until quite recently, most of the visible results in facial and skin antiaging could be achieved only with plastic surgery. Beginning in the late 1980s, however, skin researchers, who had focused primarily on treating or curing disease, began studying healthy skin and ways to improve it. Alpha-hydroxy acids were the first by-product of that research, followed by retinoids and antioxidants.

Today the profusion of treatments available at the dermatologist's office provides spot remedies so effective that women are using them to replace or at least significantly delay surgery. Some are technical and complex (Fraxel lasers and light-emitting diodes, for example). Others are so familiar they trip off the tongue like state capitals: Restylane. Collagen. Botox. Cosmeceuticals are the latest option, and the new breeds are so accessible that they are poised to democratize the once exclusive realm of the dermatologist's arsenal.

Of course, the best remedy, according to dermatologists, is a free one: prevention. "Stay out of the sun or wear sunscreen!" says Dr. Patricia Wexler of New York City, whose practice is so busy that new patients wait six months for an appointment. "My mother was my biggest influence, and she stayed out of the sun her entire life. So, at the very least, wear a big-brimmed hat!"

A New Wave in Scientific Skin Care
Make way for the cosmeceuticals

Antiaging products and skin care are the fastest-growing segments of the $200 billion-plus global beauty industry, outpacing fragrance and color cosmetics. And the demand for pretty skin is definitely on the rise. At last count there were 10,000 dermatologists in the U.S. According to the American Society for Aesthetic Plastic Surgery, 2.8 million Botox injections were given in the U.S. in 2004, a 25% increase from 2003. Chemical peels grew 54%, to more than 1.1 million.

The latest wrinkle in the long pursuit of the fountain of youth is cosmeceuticals. Make no mistake: these are not your grandmother's face cream. *Cosmeceutical* is a term for almost any cosmetic product containing ingredients capable of producing visible changes. Call them smart cosmetics. Companies from Estee Lauder, L'Oréal and Skin-Ceuticals to N.V. Perricone M.D. and Rodan + Fields are creating toners and serums and creams that claim to work less like makeup and more like medicine.

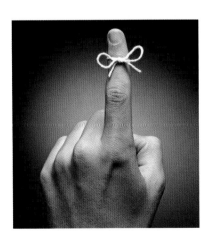

Fewer Senior Moments A major study shows that more elderly Americans are staying mentally alert

Researchers at the University of Michigan studying 11,000 elderly Americans found that people over 70 are sharper than ever. Over a nine-year period, the investigators report, the rate of significant cognitive impairment, including Alzheimer's disease and other types of dementia, declined from 12.2% of the sample population to 8.7%.

Some memory loss is inevitable with age, but the improvements shown in the study suggest that at least some lapses can be held off, in part by protecting the brain with mental stimulation and keeping the heart healthy, which enhances circulation and keeps neurons active.

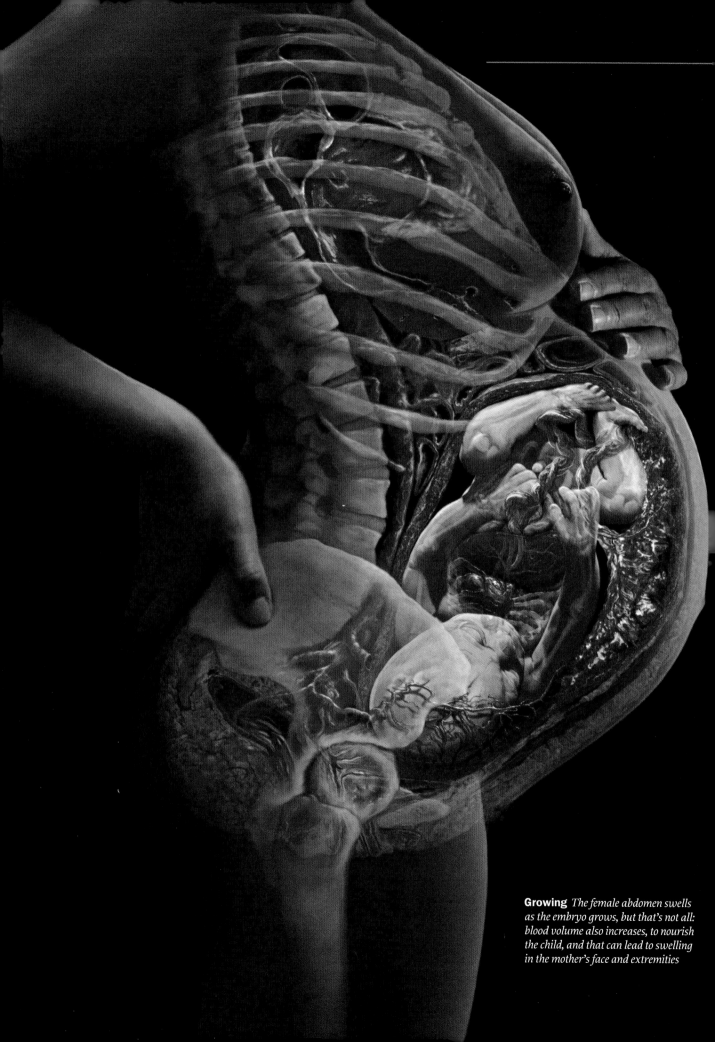

Growing *The female abdomen swells as the embryo grows, but that's not all: blood volume also increases, to nourish the child, and that can lead to swelling in the mother's face and extremities*

Creating New Life

Two journeys, one fateful meeting: the reproductive system

EVERY SYSTEM IN YOUR BODY IS DESIGNED TO ENSURE your survival, even if that survival is not about you but about your species. Reproduction in our species relies on four key operations: the generation of egg and sperm cells; fertilizing the egg; nurturing the developing offspring; and producing the proper hormones to orchestrate the entire process. Men contribute little more than DNA to the creation of a new child, so male gametes (or sperm) are small and generated by the trillions over a man's lifetime. But female gametes contain much more than just DNA: each egg cell, or ovum, is packed with nutrients and fat to nourish a growing embryo. That extra cargo makes female ova the largest cells in a human body, sometimes visible without the aid of a microscope.

Ova are also far more scarce than sperm: a woman's lifetime supply of eggs numbers only in the hundreds of thousands, compared to the millions of sperm a man can produce in a single ejaculation. Fewer than 500 of the few eggs a woman does produce will ever be released from the ovaries during ovulation and thus stand a chance of being fertilized. Both male and female gametes are fleeting: sperm cells live about 36 hours before dying, while ova are viable for less than 24 hours. But short life spans are the least of the challenges they face.

Sperm cells spring from more than half a mile of microscopic tubes contained within a man's testicles. At the moment of ejaculation, they must swim through another 15 in. of snaking conduits through the abdomen and finally to the penis. When sperm arrive in the vagina, the environment becomes even harsher: vaginal fluids are acidic, which means that sperm have to move quickly to find their target, the egg, before they are destroyed.

As if that weren't enough, the female's immune system is also on alert for the sperm, which normally would appear as foreign intruders, no different than bacteria or viruses. Here, however, the sperm at least are prepared—they come equipped with a shield of glycoprotein that allows them to sneak past the female body's immune sentries. Along the way, chemicals also change the sperm cell's surface to make it easier for the tiny sperm to be welcomed by an egg cell.

The sperm's journey up the fallopian tubes can take as much as two days. For the one-in-a-million sperm cell that survives the trip and adheres to an egg, the process of reproduction begins: the membranes of the ovum and sperm fuse into a single exterior shell, while the 23 chromosomes in the sperm and egg pair up to form a new cell, a zygote with 46 chromosomes, a complete genetic blueprint for a new person.

Egg cells are released from the woman's ovaries, which are about the size and shape of an almond, roughly every

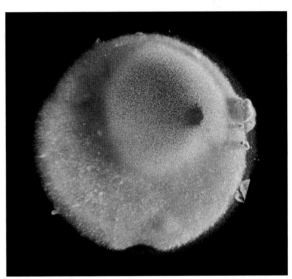

Female egg *This oocyte cell has not yet fully matured; its nucleus is the red sphere at center*

28 days, then journey down the fallopian tubes, or oviducts, to the uterus. Sperm cells generally find their egg targets for fertilization in the oviducts. But whether or not an egg is fertilized, it embeds itself in the uterine wall after its journey through the tubes. Unfertilized eggs are then flushed from the uterus, along with the entire uterine wall, during menstruation. A fertilized egg, however, remains firmly in place, and begins to absorb nourishment from the blood vessels of the richly endowed uterus; over the course of the next 40 weeks, it will grow into a human baby. ∎

■ **Anatomy Lesson** The Reproductive System

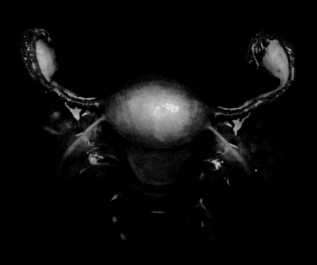

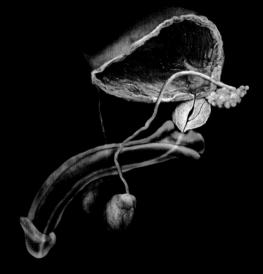

Internal organs *The two ovaries, fallopian tubes, uterus, cervix and vagina are the principal female reproductive organs*

Internal/external organs *The male's penis and testes are outside the torso; prostate and epididymis are inside*

The Female System

The female reproductive system does the lion's share of the work in procreation: it manufactures and nurtures the egg cell and moves it from the ovaries to the fallopian tubes, where fertilization usually takes place. It then provides the environment in which the fertilized egg can develop into a fetus and, about 270 days later, a full-term baby.

The exquisitely engineered system that accomplishes these many tasks includes the ovaries, which produce egg cells, and the fallopian tubes that connect the ovaries to the uterus, a hollow, internal chamber of muscle where fertilized eggs grow into fully developed embryos. Beneath the uterus lies the cervix, a narrow passageway that leads to the vagina, a 4-in. long muscular tunnel that discharges menstrual flow and serves as the birth canal during labor.

The vagina leads to the portion of the female reproductive system visible on the exterior of the body—the genitalia. These include the mons pubis (the swelling area below the stomach covered by pubic hair); two folds of skin called labia, which form the "lips" of the vagina; and the clitoris, a small erectile organ, similar to the penis, that responds to sexual stimulation. All of these converge at the external opening of the vagina, which also contains the urethra, the duct for urination.

The Male System

Male reproductive engineering is mostly external. It begins with a pair of testicles that manufacture sperm; they hang outside the torso in a saclike scrotum. These are critical to sperm production, which requires a temperature three to five degrees below that of body temperature.

After leaving the testicles, sperm passes through a looping series of internal ducts. The epididymis is a coiled tube, 18 ft. long, in which the immature sperm cells complete development to fertilize egg cells. This tube leads to the ductus deferens (also called vas deferens), which stores viable sperm and connects the epididymis to the prostate gland, a walnut-sized organ that supplies an alkaline fluid to enhance sperm motility. On the far side of the prostate gland, an ejaculatory duct leads from the prostate to the urethra, a tube that carries sperm to the tip of the penis.

Near the base of the penis are the Cowper's glands, a pair of pea-size organs that secrete an alkaline, mucus-like fluid that neutralizes the acidity of any urine residue in the urethra, which could harm sperm. The penis itself consists of three columns of spongy erectile tissue that fill with blood and become rigid when sexually excited. The penis is tipped with the glans, which contains a small slit through which sperm (and urine) urine exit the body.

Common Reproductive Diseases and Disorders

Chlamydia The most common sexually transmitted disease (STD), it can lead to pelvic inflammatory disease and infertility.

■ **Symptoms** *Men: discharge from penis or rectum, burning on urination or defecation. Women: vaginal discharge, burning on urination, pain during sexual intercourse or abdominal pain. In 25-30% of cases there are no symptoms.*

■ **Treatment** Antibiotics—for both partners.

Genital Herpes A sexually transmitted viral infection that affects the skin of the genitals.

■ **Symptoms** *Eruptions of small, painful blisters filled with clear, straw-colored fluid in the genital area. Fever, malaise, muscle aches.*

■ **Treatment** There is no cure. Antiviral medications can relieve the symptoms and shorten healing time. Daily medications can prevent recurrence.

Gonorrhea A sexually transmitted infection caused by bacteria.

■ **Symptoms** *Discharge from penis or vagina; for women, bleeding during*

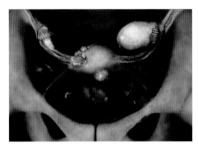

Uterine intruders *Cysts, fibroids and teratomas, above, can afflict the uterus. They are benign but can be very painful and interfere with pregnancy*

intercourse, painful urination.

■ **Treatment** Antibiotics. Use of a condom reduces but does not eliminate chances of infection.

Pelvic Inflammatory Disease Infection and inflammation of the lining of the uterus, the fallopian tubes or the ovaries, often as a result of sexual contact. Can lead to infertility or ectopic pregnancy.

■ **Symptoms** *Vaginal discharge, abdominal pain, fever.*

■ **Treatment** Antibiotics; intravenous antibiotics for severe cases.

Gardasil for Girls?

It's one of the most heated public-health matters of the moment: vaccinating tweenage girls against a sexually transmitted virus long before they become sexually active. Gardasil, approved by the FDA in 2007, protects against four strains of

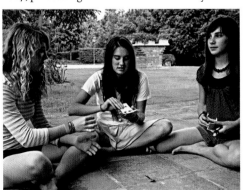

human papillomavirus (HPV). Two are believed to cause 70% of cases of cervical cancer. The other two strains cause 90% of genital warts cases. Studies show about 40% of girls become infected with HPV within two years of becoming sexually active.

Many parents are deeply uncomfortable with the vaccination, feeling it is an invitation to begin premature sexual activity. In 2007, after Texas Governor Rick Perry tried and failed to make the vaccination mandatory for sixth-grade girls, maker Merck stopped lobbying states to require the vaccine for school.

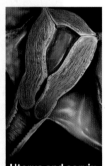

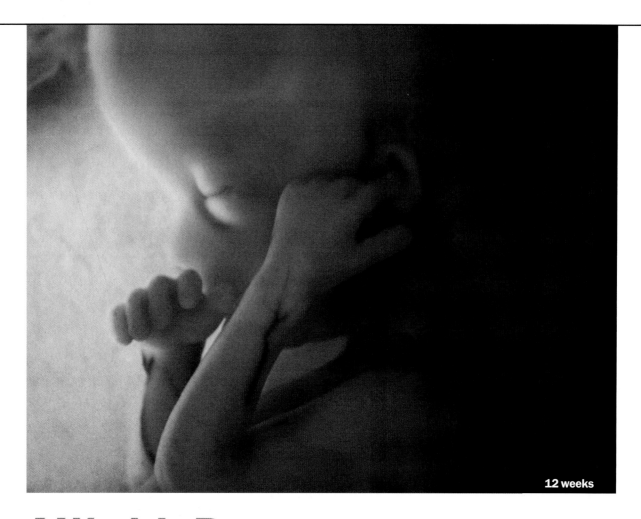

12 weeks

A Work in Progress Stages of fetal development

HUMANS FIRST PEERED INTO THE WOMB THANKS TO the groundbreaking photography of Lennart Nilsson, whose pictures of the development of the fetus caused a sensation when published in LIFE magazine in 1965. Thanks to today's powerful imaging technologies, we are more familiar than ever with the stages of fetal growth and development, yet the process remains astonishing. After the genetic material from the egg and sperm merge to form a new, unique cell that shares the chromosomes of both mother and father, development is rapid. In its earliest stage, the embryo resembles a salamander or tadpole, complete with a tail rather than legs. But within weeks the hallmarks of a human begin to form: arms and legs, a beating heart, a brain whose neurons are multiplying and forming synapses.

At four weeks the embryo is about the size of a pea; at eight weeks it is the size of a large grape; at 12 weeks it is the size of a lemon and is referred to as a fetus. Throughout the pregnancy, the fetus draws all its nourishment from its mother. In its early days, the embryo is nourished by a yolk sac that grows richer with blood vessels until it forms a placenta that attaches to the uterine wall. The embryo and placenta are connected by an umbilical cord, through which the fetus is nourished and its waste products are removed.

The baby's head appears large and out of proportion to the rest of the body well into the pregnancy, an indication of its primacy among the body's organs. At 12 weeks, the end of the first trimester of pregnancy, the fetus can clearly be seen as a human being; it has toes and fingers, two eyes (fused shut for safety), and it can open and close its mouth. The major internal organs are recognizable, but the immune, endocrine and other advanced systems are still developing.

The final two trimesters of pregnancy are devoted primarily to the growth of the fetus rather than its development. Now it is the mother's turn to experience major body changes, as the growing fetus swells her abdomen, her heart beats faster to provide more blood to the fetus, and her growing uterus presses upon and shrinks her bladder, with predictable results. In most cases, the final preparation for birth finds the fetus turning within the uterus so that its head will face the birth canal, ready for its passage from the womb into the larger world. ■

First trimester *At 12 weeks, above, one-third of the way through the pregnancy, the fingers of the fetus are clearly formed*

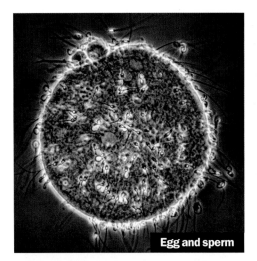

Egg and sperm

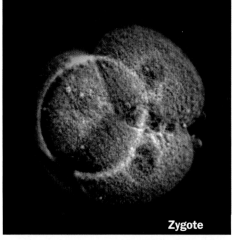

Zygote

Conception *At left, sperm cells surround the much larger egg, attempting to breach its membranes. Only one will succeed and fuse its genetic material with that of the egg.*

At right, conception has taken place, the cells have fused, and a zygote has formed and has begun dividing into additional cells.

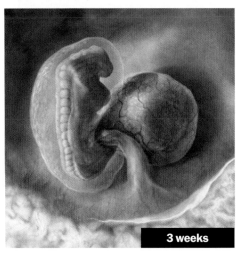

3 weeks

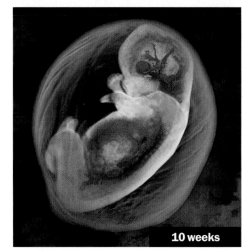

10 weeks

Early days *In its first nine weeks, the embryo depends on the yolk sac, the orb at right in the left picture, for nourishment. This sac later develops into the placenta that nourishes the fetus. At 10 weeks, the fetus, now 2 in. long, floats in an amniotic sac, and internal structures are beginning to take definite form.*

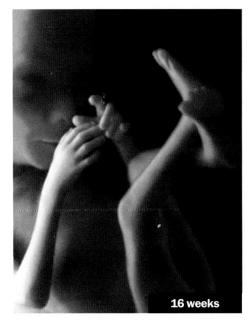

16 weeks

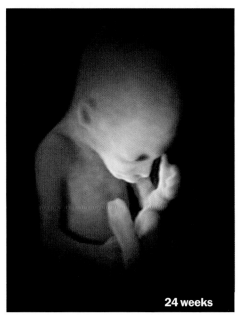

24 weeks

Growing *At 16 weeks, the fetus is 3.5 to 6 in. long The body has begun to elongate, as neck and back muscles develop and spine, rib cage and shoulders knit together and harden. Eight weeks later, the right ear is beginning to form; the eyes are closed, with fused eyelids. The fetus may now be 10 in. long.*

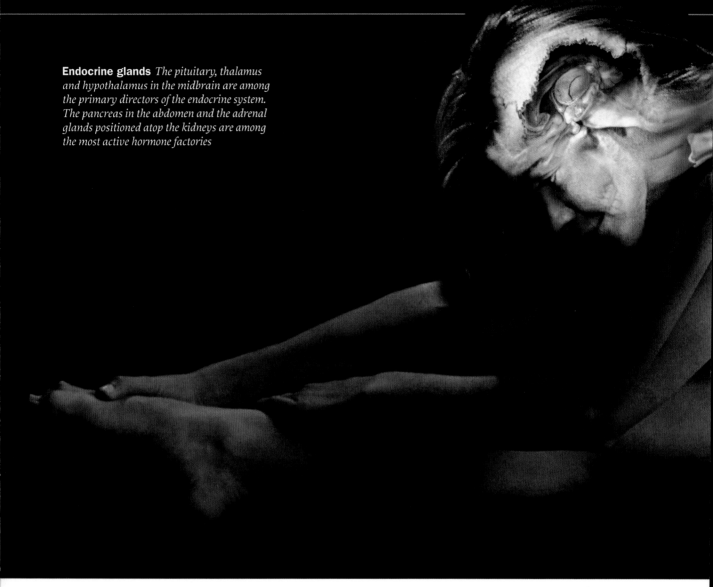

Endocrine glands *The pituitary, thalamus and hypothalamus in the midbrain are among the primary directors of the endocrine system. The pancreas in the abdomen and the adrenal glands positioned atop the kidneys are among the most active hormone factories*

Chemical Communicators
Hormones are the body's unsung messengers

AN AMAZING NETWORK OF NERVES COMMANDS THE body's communications system, yet there is another set of intricately connected organs and cells that are critical to ensuring that your food is digested, that your cells continue to grow and that you are able to reproduce. It's a system that relies on chemicals rather than electrical impulses, and whose effects, if less immediate than a muscle twitch, can have a far more lasting influence on our lives. This is the endocrine network, which sends a cascade of chemical messengers called hormones flooding through the bloodstream. Sometimes triggered in a flash in response to immediate stimuli like fear, hunger or sexual arousal, the endocrine system also initiates long-term changes in our life cycle, switching on the reproductive system during puberty or

turning it off decades later, at menopause. And it's not just the hormones themselves that take up the call, but also the network of glands throughout the body that produces them, as well as the specialized receptors that recognize and respond to them.

Our endocrine glands produce about 50 different hormones, all of which fall into two broad categories: peptides, which are protein-based, and steroids, which are made of fatty material. The vast majority of human hormones are peptides. Steroids are produced only by the reproductive and adrenal glands. Peptides and steroids perform a wide array of functions, from maintaining the body's metabolism moment by moment (working in tandem with the nervous system) to regulating growth (a process in which the nervous system plays

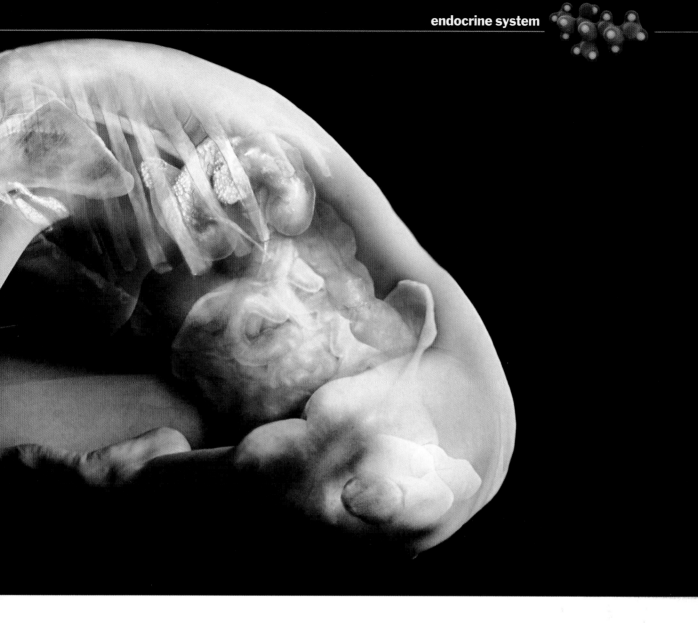

almost no role, and the endocrine system is dominant).

The pancreas exerts an important influence in both the endocrine and digestive systems, while the testes and ovaries are central to the functioning of the reproductive system. Yet even among the hard-working organs of this network, the pituitary, located on the underside of the brain, stands alone. It is the pituitary that secretes hormones that control most of the other endocrine glands. Among these are the hypothalamus, also located beneath the brain, which plays an important role as a conduit between the endocrine and nervous systems.

While messages carried by the nervous system act a bit like a telegraph, bouncing between the brain and a specific point elsewhere in the body, the endocrine system functions more like a bullhorn: its message is carried far and wide, until it is picked up by the intended audience of cells. To make sure the signal gets to the right recipients (and only the right recipients), every molecule of a hormone is encased in proteins that fit perfectly into grooves on the surface of receptor cells, much as a key can slide only into a specific lock.

If the amount and mixture of hormones in the bloodstream are not tightly regulated, many essential body processes would spin out of control. The system monitors itself by negative feedback: when cells or organs targeted by a hormone from the thyroid gland, for example, shift into overdrive, a new signal travels back to the hypothalamus, which sends a message to the pituitary to stop secreting the hormone that originally spurred the thyroid into action. ∎

Anatomy Lesson The Endocrine System

The master manipulator of the endocrine system is the pituitary gland, a pea-sized organ that sits above the spine and beneath the brain. Linked to the brain and the nervous system via the hypothalamus, it pumps out hormones that regulate other endocrine organs, especially the thyroid, adrenal and reproductive glands. It's the pituitary that also releases hormones that act directly on the bones, kidneys and the uterus. Situated slightly above and behind the pituitary is the pineal gland, a cone-shaped organ that produces the hormone melatonin, which helps control reproductive development in both sexes, as well as daily metabolism and sleep cycles.

A few inches below these glands, in the neck, are the thyroid and parathyroid glands. The bow tie–shaped thyroid straddles the trachea and produces hormones that regulate the rate at which the body burns food to create energy. It plays an expanded role during childhood, helping to orchestrate development in the bones, brain and nervous system.

Further down the body are the adrenal glands: twin, triangular organs positioned atop each kidney. Their cortex, or outer layer, maintains the saline levels of tissues in the body, monitors metabolism and the immune system, influences sexual development and fuels the body's response to stress. Embedded inside the cortex is the medulla, which secretes adrenaline, the biological super-fuel that accelerates the heart rate and blood pressure into a fight-or-flight state.

Between the kidneys is the pancreas, which secretes vital juices for the digestive system and also produces two hormones, insulin and glucagon, that together maintain the right amount of sugar in the blood; when they don't, diabetes sets in.

The endocrine system also controls the essential process of reproduction. The gonads are gender-specific glands that produce hormones to regulate the body's sexual development. Male testes make testosterone, while female ovaries secrete estrogen, responsible for the maturing of sexual characteristics, and progesterone, responsible for the thickening of the lining of the uterus each month.

Not to be outdone by these primary organs, other structures of the body can secrete hormones: the mucosa that line the digestive tract, for example, secrete hormones important to digestion. The heart also churns out atriopeptin, a blood-pressure regulator. The brain, lungs, kidneys, liver and skin also produce hormones to keep their daily operations running smoothly.

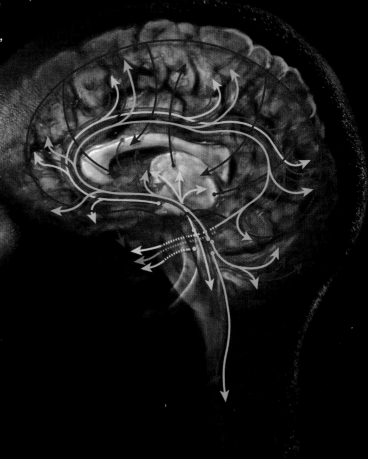

Pathways *Like the hormones of the endocrine system, neurotransmitters are chemical messengers concentrated in the brain but active throughout th entire body*

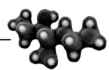

Endocrine System Diseases and Disorders

Addison's Disease Occurs when the adrenal glands produce too few corticosteroids, usually due to damage to the adrenal cortex from autoimmune disease, infections (such as tuberculosis, HIV or fungal infections), hemorrhage or blood loss.

▥ **Symptoms** *Changes in blood pressure or heart rate, chronic diarrhea, darkening of the skin, paleness, extreme weakness, fatigue, appetite loss, nausea and vomiting, salt craving, slow or sluggish movement.*

▥ **Treatment** Replacement corticosteroids can control the symptoms but usually need to be taken for life.

Diabetes A life-long disease marked by high levels of sugar in the blood, usually caused by too little insulin (the hormone that controls blood sugar), resistance to insulin (in which muscle, fat and liver cells do not respond to it) or both.

▥ **Symptoms** *For Type 1 diabetes (too little insulin): increased thirst and urination; weight loss in spite of greater appetite; fatigue; nausea; and vomiting.*
For Type 2 (insulin resistance): increased thirst, urination and appetite; fatigue; blurred vision; slow-healing infections.

▥ **Treatment** Incurable, but medication, diet and exercise programs can control blood-sugar levels and prevent complications.

Goiter Noncancerous enlargement of the thyroid gland due to under-production of thyroid hormone, often due to lack of iodine in the diet, causing swelling.

▥ **Symptoms** *A swollen thyroid can exert pressure on the windpipe and esophagus, leading to breathing difficulties, coughing, swallowing difficulties and wheezing.*

▥ **Treatment** Radioactive iodine to shrink the gland, surgery to remove all or part of the gland, iodine doses to reduce deficiency.

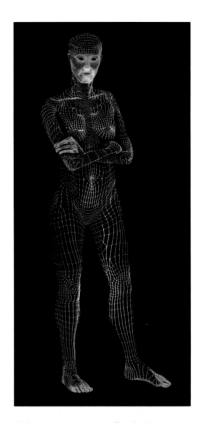

The Endocrine System Terms to Know

Acromegaly Excessive growth due to overproduction of growth hormone by the pituitary gland.

Corticosteroids Hormones produced by the adrenal gland, consisting of hydrocortisone and corticosterone; involved in stress, immune response, metabolism and inflammation.

Estrogen/Progesterone Hormones secreted by the ovaries that affect many aspects of the female body, including menstrual cycles and pregnancy.

Hormone A chemical created by the body that controls numerous body functions.

Insulin A hormone released by the pancreas that regulates sugar use in the body.

Islets of Langerhans Pancreatic cells that produce insulin and glucagon, important regulators of sugar metabolism.

Oxytocin A hormone secreted by the pituitary gland that plays a role in childbirth and lactation in new mothers.

Thyroid Endocrine gland that straddles the trachea and produces hormones that regulate metabolism.

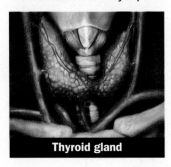

Thyroid gland

Sources (2): University of Virginia Health System, University of Maryland Medical Center

Pheromones Subtle, silent signals

Pheromones are among the body's more fascinating chemical communicators. Unlike hormones, which regulate activity within the body itself, pheromones are designed to trigger responses in another member of the same species. These signaling devices are heavily used by insects, animals and even plants, which rely on pheromones to sound an alarm, to attract a mate or to signal food trails.

The illustration above shows the areas of pheromone production in the human body, with the most active areas appearing in red. In humans, pheromones appear to work through the sense of smell, and some research suggests that pheromones are responsible for synchronizing menstrual cycles among women living in close proximity. But cosmetics claiming to contain pheromones acting as aphrodisiacs are more sniff than science.

■ On the Horizon Briefs

Teens Before Their Time Girls are growing up earlier than ever—but why?

Growing old is not something that most of us look forward to, but when you're a teenager, there's nothing you yearn for more than to look mature for your years. And It seems as if everywhere you turn these days—outside schools, on soccer fields, at the mall—girls are developing faster than they ever have, both socially and biologically. It's as if an entire generation of girls has been put on fast-forward: filling out and growing up all in a rush. The first major scientific paper on the subject, published in 1997, showed that significant numbers of white girls—some 15%—were showing outward signs of incipient sexual maturity by age 8, and about 5% as early as 7. Among African-American girls, 15% were developing breasts or pubic hair by age 7, and almost half by age 8.

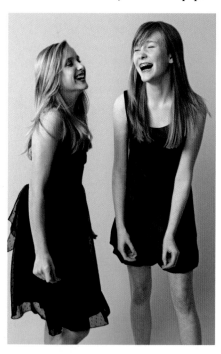

What's going on? Is it something in the water? Scientists are struggling to nail down a cause, but they do have a long list of potential theories. The leading candidate? That early puberty is somehow tied up with a much more familiar phenomenon: America's obesity epidemic. Some scientists suspect that early breast development may be encouraged by a protein called leptin, which is produced by fat cells and is essential to the onset of puberty. Another clue comes from the fact that overweight girls have more insulin circulating in their blood, which may stimulate the production of sex hormones from the ovary and the adrenal gland.

If it's not obesity, other researchers argue, the chemicals that today's girls are exposed to could play a role. DDE, for example, a breakdown product of the pesticide DDT, and PCBS, once used as flame retardants in electrical equipment, are known to be endocrine disruptors. Others point to an ingredient in plastics, phthalates, which has been shown to cause birth defects and change hormone levels in rats; studies on humans are ongoing. Regardless of the cause, however, parents and doctors should be aware that sexual maturation isn't just physical; the changes in the body come along with psychological consequences that still-developing girls may need extra help to handle

The Chemistry of Desire How biochemicals turn us on

Human sexuality is a maze in which mind, body and experience are endlessly intermingled. People find themselves aroused in obvious situations—slow-dancing together, seeing someone with a sexy body. But carnal longings strike at surprising times too—even after a tragedy, like the death of a parent.

No matter how lust is triggered, though, sex, like eating or sleeping, is governed by biochemicals that interact in complicated ways to create the familiar sensations of desire, arousal, orgasm. And over the past decade or two, scientists have identified many of the pieces of this complex puzzle.

Desire clearly involves testosterone—in both men and women—along with other hormones, including estrogen and oxytocin, which is intimately connected with female sexualilty and menstruation. But increasingly, scientists are exploring the action of neurotransmitters, chemicals that help shape our moods, emotions and attitudes. And the most central of these for the feeling we call desire seems to be dopamine, which is at least partly responsible for making external stimuli arousing. Another neurotransmitter, serotonin, pairs with dopamine to create the complicated feelings of desire.

Scientists have also learned that the old notion that 90% of sex is in the mind is literally true: parts of the brain involved in sexual response include the basal ganglia, the anterior insula cortex, the amygdala, the cerebellum and the hypothalamus.

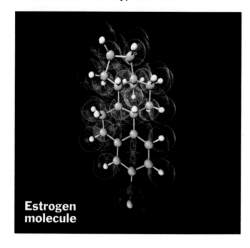

Estrogen molecule

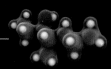

■ Briefing Hormones and Neurotransmitters

Biochemistry is producing some of our most illuminating insights into the way that compounds such as hormones and neurotransmitters direct critical functions in the body, from sexual arousal to behavior. Sophisticated new technologies such as positron-emission tomography (PET), which allows scientists to record brain activity in real time, are revealing which areas of the brain are recruited to activate specific moods, memories and perceptions.

Biochemists have long known that many of the body's processes are directed by the hormones secreted by the pituitary gland and other organs of the endocrine system. But increasingly they are recognizing the contribution of neurotransmitters, the chemicals of the nervous system generated in the brain that play a role in many of our daily activities: desire, sleep, memory, pain, anger. Much like hormones, neurotransmitters operate across the body; they are released at the synapses of nerve cells, or neurons, and keep the impulses flowing along the body's network of nerves. The table below shows only a fraction of the more significant of the body's many chemical messengers, but it demonstrates the powerful roles biochemicals play in our lives.

Hormones and Neurotransmitters

Dopamine Studies show that the levels of this neurotransmitter are highly correlated with the level of desire. Dopamine-producing neurons in the central part of the brain color one's perception of the outside world, creating what is experienced as a sexy mood. And because of its connection to feelings of satisfaction, it may also drive some people to form powerful attachments to drugs, alcohol, smoking and other addictive behaviors.

Epinephrine and Norepinephrine These substances play dual roles as hormones and neurotransmitters. Both are involved with stress reactions, including the fight-or-flight response.

Estrogen A hormone produced in the ovaries and the brain that regulates ovulation, it's also involved in creating feelings of desire in both men and women, possibly by stimulating the release of dopamine.

GABA Considered a primary neurotransmitter that broadly affects most brain neurons, Gamma-aminobutyric acts as the body's neural brake, suppressing or shutting down communication between neurons. It may also modulate the action of other neurotransmitters such as dopamine

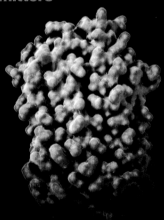

Norepeniphrine molecule

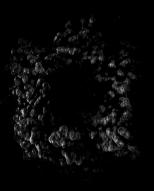

GABA molecule

and serotonin. And it helps regulate muscle tone. Abnormal levels of GABA may be behind such neurological disorders as epilepsy and spastic cerebral palsy, in which signals to motor nerves fail to fire properly.

Oxytocin A hormone released by the pituitary gland, ovaries and testes, it helps to activate milk production and uterine contractions during childbirth. It also plays a role in establishing the emotional bond between parents and their children. Studies show that levels of oxytocin rise in men when their partners become pregnant.

Serotonin This neurotransmitter is produced in the midbrain and brain stem and is the key to satisfaction. Serotonin can increase sexual desire—most likely by working in concert with dopamine—but only to a certain extent. Drugs like Prozac that boost serotonin levels can also make orgasm harder to achieve.

Testosterone Small quantities of this hormone are made in the brain, but most of it is produced in the testes and ovaries; in women it is quickly converted into estrogen. For men, it's the key hormone of desire, creating feelings of positive energy and well-being. When it's depleted, both men and women experience low libido.

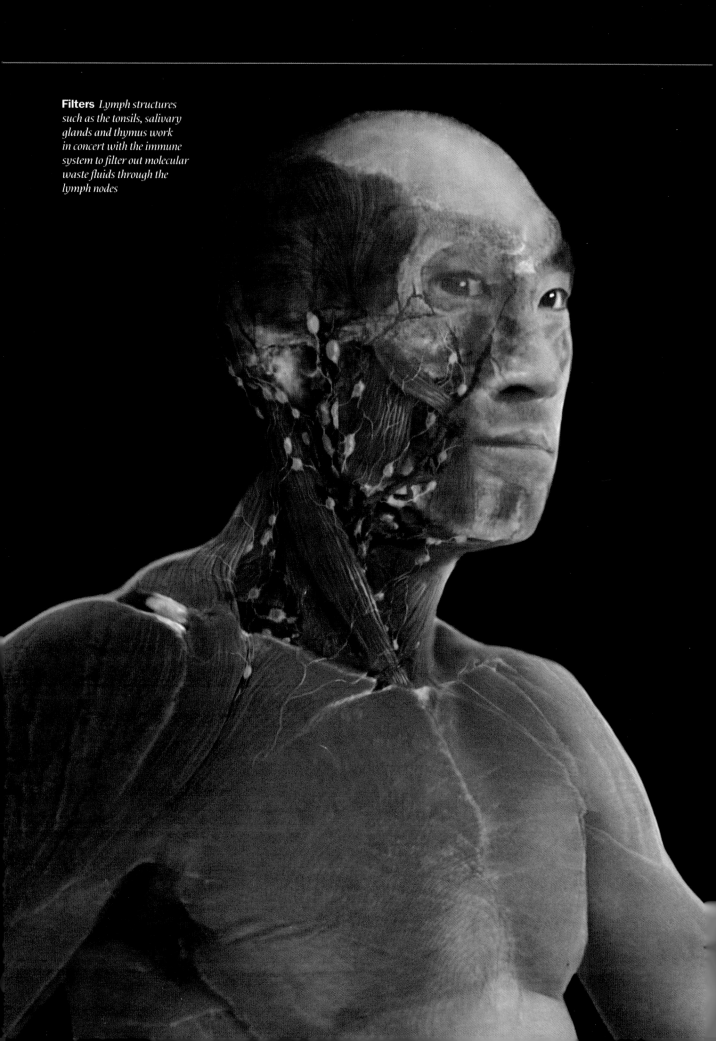

Filters *Lymph structures such as the tonsils, salivary glands and thymus work in concert with the immune system to filter out molecular waste fluids through the lymph nodes*

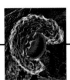

Defensive Perimeter

Seek, identify, contact, destroy: the immune system

LIFE IS OFTEN HARSH FOR THE BACTERIA, VIRUSES and other pathogens that are found almost everywhere in nature. Small wonder, then, that they seek the ideal environment to escape the heat, cold, dehydration, starvation and ruthless predation of the world: your body. Every day of your life, you are the target of round-the-clock assaults and invasions: at any given moment, your skin resembles a Normandy beach on D-day.

Nature's answer to this constant state of siege is the immune system, a network of cells, tissues and organs

stroy; and, finally, killing disease-causing bugs directly.

The third shield is the adaptive, or "acquired," system, which is trained to identify and kill particular bacteria or viruses. The adaptive immune system's power lies in its ability to remember old enemies and thus shorten the time it takes to dispatch the proper killing forces against repeat-invaders—a skill feature known as active immunity. Passive immunity, on the other hand, comes from co-opting an existing set of already-marshalled biological defenses—such as an unborn baby's immune responses,

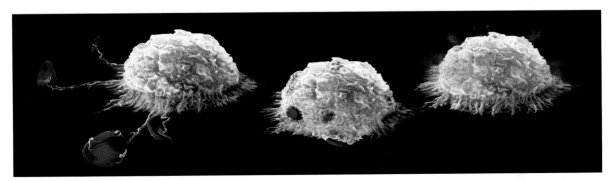

On patrol *Besides repelling intruders, the immune system helps police the body; here a macrophage weeds out old red blood cells*

that cooperate to defend the body in two ways: by keeping foreign intruders out whenever possible and by hunting down and killing those that slip through its arsenal of defensive weapons. First, there are physical barriers to invasion—the skin; the sticky, mucous fluids that cover openings like the mouth; and the tiny hairs that line passages leading from the outside world to your body's interior. The acids in your stomach are another obstacle, able to burn most bacteria that hitch a ride inside your body aboard food.

The second line of defense is the innate immune system, which takes a blanket approach to identifying any foreign substance within the body and destroying it. These responses include inflammation, which creates temporary physical barriers at the site of the invasion; summoning macrophages to the scene to devour invaders; enveloping intruders to make them easier to de-

which come from its mother. This type of immunity, however, is only short term and remains only for as long as the borrowed defenses remain in the bloodstream.

How does the immune system know friend from foe? Nearly every cell in your body carries a code, a protein password on its surface that tells your immune system to ignore it. Intruding cells, or antigens, carry different markers that quickly set off alarms. Should this strategy fail, and your system lose the ability to distinguish "self" from "non-self," it can attack itself, which occurs in autoimmune diseases such as lupus or arthritis.

On a much less threatening scale, your protective system can misfire and go on "red alert" over a harmless antigen, such as pollen, which most of us will recognize as an allergy. *Ah-choo!* ∎

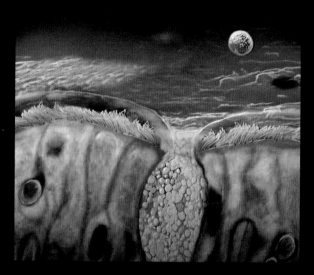
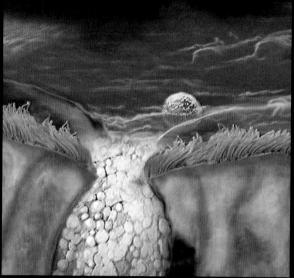
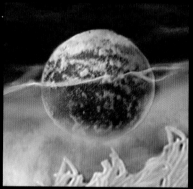
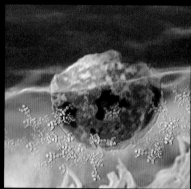

Apprehended and dispatched
The immune system operates in a wide variety of forms, marshaling an array of defensive weapons. This sequence shows a disease-carrying microbe trapped by the microscopic hairs along the mucous membrane of the nose. Once ensnared, the invading microbe is recognized and attacked by enzymes manufactured to hunt and seek such intruders. In the last illustration, the enzymes have begun to degrade the bacterium

■ Anatomy Lesson The Immune System

The next time you fight off a cold, or make it through a bout with the flu, you can thank your immune system. Between the white blood cells coursing through arteries and veins and the lymphatic system, which drains and cleanses tissues of toxins, your body has a pretty good system for protecting cells from infection.

White blood cells are the foundation of human immunity. They are manufactured by bone marrow, then pass directly into the bloodstream as phagocytes and granulocytes. Phagocytes are designed to engulf and digest anything that doesn't belong in the bloodstream, while granulocytes contain tiny granules filled with toxins that can poison unwelcome cells. Some phagocytes also act as molecular town criers, secreting chemicals called cytokines that call for additional help, even as they are launching the first wave of attack on invading bugs. Other phagocytic cells transport the remains of an intruder back to lymph nodes, where they can be logged for future identification. White blood cells are indiscriminate killers: they target anything that does not look biologically familiar.

While these white blood cells are at work, other immune cells migrate to the lymph system, where they evolve into a variety of specialized hunter-killer cells, each designed to recognize and destroy a specific kind of foreign invader. These lymphocytes fall into two major categories: B cells (which take their abbreviation from bone, where they mature) and T cells (which reach full potency in the thymus).

In the simplest terms, these security agents divvy up the dirty work of immunity. B cells find and identify the bad guys, after which T cells destroy them. When an invasion has been repelled, some of the B cells and T cells that were involved in the battle morph into specialized "memory cells" and remain in the body for many years. Their job is to scan for the same intruder and launch the same chemical defense strategy as the first time around—but this time, because they have seen the invaders before, they are hopefully able to respond sooner and with more force. Memory cells like these make it possible for us to suffer from some diseases, chicken pox for example, only once.

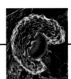

Common Immune System Diseases and Disorders

AIDS (Acquired Immunodeficiency Syndrome) The most advanced stage of HIV (human immunodeficiency virus) infection causes severe damage to the immune system, leaving the patient essentially unprotected from infection of any kind.

■ **Symptoms** *Numerous and varied, they are primarily the result of opportunistic infections that individuals with a healthy immune system can easily overcome, including fevers, night sweats, swollen glands, chills, weakness and weight loss.*

■ **Treatment** AIDS is currently

cans more than those of other races). Lupus causes inflammation of the skin, joints, kidneys and other organs.

■ **Symptoms** *Joint pain (especially in extremities) and arthritis. Inflammation of parts of the heart is common, as are chest pain and arrhythmias. General symptoms include fever, fatigue, malaise, skin rash, swollen glands, muscle aches, nausea and vomiting.*

■ **Treatment** Lupus is incurable, and treatment is designed to control symptoms. Mild cases require little therapy; severe or life-threatening

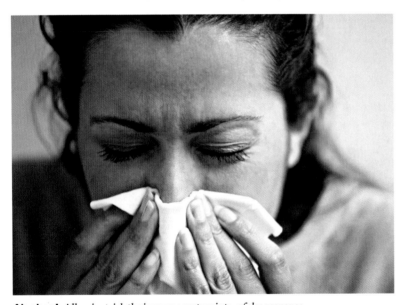

Ah-choo! *Allergies trick the immune system into a false response*

incurable, but a variety of treatments can help keep symptoms at bay and improve the quality of life of those who are infected. Antiretroviral drugs suppress the replication of the HIV virus. A mix of these agents, highly active antiretroviral therapy (HAART), is very effective in reducing the number of HIV particles in the bloodstream. But HAART has complications and side effects, and the virus can develop resistance to the drugs, requiring the use of alternate drug combinations.

Lupus Systemic lupus erythematosus is an autoimmune disease in which the body attacks its own tissues. It affects women far more often than men (and African Ameri-

cases often require treatment by a rheumatologist. Corticosteroids or other medications may be used.

Rheumatoid Arthritis An autoimmune disease in which joints and surrounding tissues become chronically inflamed.

■ **Symptoms** *Fatigue, morning stiffness, widespread muscle aches, loss of appetite, weakness. Often followed by joint pain and swelling and by destruction of the joint.*

■ **Treatment** Medications, physical therapy, exercise and surgery in extreme cases. Early, aggressive treatment can delay deterioration of the joint.

Source: National Institutes of Health

Source: National Institutes of Health

Immune System Terms to Know

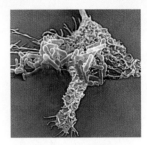

Cleanup *A macrophage (purple) ingests bacteria*

Allergic diseases Those that trigger a false alarm in the immune system, causing it to treat common, harmless allergens like pet hair and pollen as a threat.

Antibody A molecule produced by a mature B cell that is designed to specifically recognize and attach to an allergen. Also called an immunoglobulin.

Bacterium A single-celled organism, many of which can carry disease.

Inflammation An immune system reaction to foreign invaders such as microbes or allergens. Signs include redness, swelling, pain or heat, as increased blood flow sends an influx of immune cells to the site.

Macrophage A large and versatile immune cell that devours invading pathogens and other intruders.

Mast cell A granulocyte found in tissue that triggers allergic reactions.

Pathogen An organism or virus that causes disease.

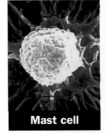

Mast cell

Source: National Institute of Allergy and Infectious Diseases

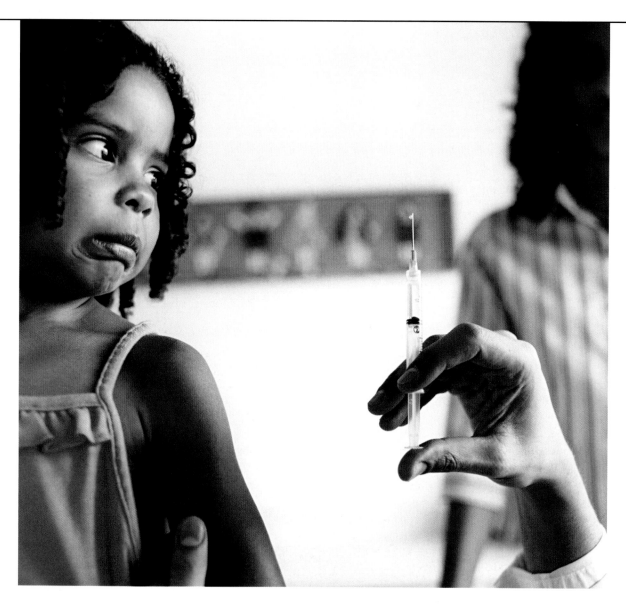

How Safe Are Vaccines?

Morе parents are declining the shots—but is that the right decision?

EVER SINCE EDWARD JENNER, A COUNTRY DOCTOR IN England, inoculated his son and a handful of other children against smallpox in 1796 by exposing them to cowpox pus, things have been tougher on humans' most unwelcome intruders, the bacteria and viruses that cause infectious disease. In the past century, vaccines against diphtheria, polio, pertussis, measles, mumps and rubella, not to mention the more recent additions of hepatitis B and chickenpox, have wired humans with powerful immune sentries to ward off uninvited invasions. And thanks to state laws requiring vaccinations for youngsters enrolling in kindergarten, the U.S. currently enjoys the highest immunization rate ever: 77% of children embarking on the first day of school are completely up to date on their recommended shots.

Yet simmering beneath these national numbers is a trend that's working in the microbes' favor—and against ours. Spurred by claims that vaccinations can be linked to autism, parents in increasing numbers are raising questions about whether vaccines, far from panaceas, are actually harmful to children. When the immune system of a baby or young child is just coming online, is it such a good idea to challenge it with antigens to so many bugs? Have the safety, efficacy and side effects of this flood of inoculations really been worked through? More and more, all this wrangling over risks and benefits is leading confused parents to simply opt out of vaccines altogether. Despite the rules requiring students to be vaccinated, doctors can issue waivers to kids whose compromised immune system might make vaccines risky.

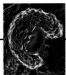

Recommended Childhood Immunization Schedule

Vaccine	Doses	At birth	1 to 2 months	2 months	4 months	6 months	6 to 18 months	6 months or older	12 to 15 months	12 to 23 months	15 to 18 months	18 months or older	4 to 6 years	11 to 12 years	Protects against
Hepatitis B	3	■	■				■								Hepatitis B (chronic inflammation of the liver)
DTaP	5			■	■	■						■	■		Diphtheria, tetanus and pertussis (whooping cough)
Hib	4			■	■	■			■						Infections of the blood, brain (meningitis), joints, inner ears or lungs (pneumonia)
Polio	4			■	■	■							■		Polio
PCV7	4			■	■	■			■						Infections of the blood, brain (meningitis), joints, inner ears or lungs (pneumonia)
Rotavirus	3			■	■	■									Rotavirus (diarrhea and vomiting)
Influenza	2†							■ ■							Flu and complications
MMR	2								■				■		Measles, mumps and rubella (German measles)
Varicella	2								■				■		Chicken pox
Hepatitis A	2									■		■			Hepatitis A (inflammation of the liver)
Tdap	1													■	Diphtheria, tetanus and pertussis (whooping cough)
MCV4	1													■	Infections of the blood, brain (meningitis), joints or lungs (pneumonia)
HPV	3													■ ■ ■	Human papillomavirus (females only)

A child can safely receive all vaccines recommended for a particular age during one visit. Combination vaccines can be used to reduce the number of injections.

*State-reported data compiled by the CDC/National Center for Immunization and Respiratory Diseases, Immunization Services Division, Assessment Branch †One dose yearly thereafter   Source: CDC

Additionally, all but two states allow waivers for children whose parents object to vaccines for religious reasons, while 20 allow parents to opt out on philosophical grounds. Currently, nearly one-half of 1% of kids enrolled in school are unvaccinated under a medical waiver, 2% to 3% have a nonmedical one, and the numbers appear to be rising.

Parents of these unimmunized kids know that as long as nearly all the other children get their shots, there should not be enough pathogen around to sicken anyone. But that's a fragile shield. Infectious-disease bugs continue to travel the globe, always ready to launch the next big public-health threat.

Public-health officials know that the only defense against the dark power of rumor is an illuminating dose of solid facts. Many of those rumors linking autism to vaccinations, for example, were sparked by a controversial British research paper published in 1998—and 10 of its 13 authors have now retracted its hypothesis. In 2003 a committee impaneled by top U.S. health officials concluded there was no scientific evidence to support such a link. Instead the panel recommended that studies focus on less explored genetic or biological explanations for the disorder. And those stories that vaccines contain too much mercury? Yes, they once did, but the U.S. government ordered all vaccines reformulated with reduced or no mercury in 2001. To vaccinate yourself against other such rumors, consult the panel at right. ■

What You Need to Know

Uncertainty over the need for and safety of vaccines widely recommended during childhood is fueling fear and confusion. Here are some answers:

Are vaccinations necessary?
Absolutely. Immunizing all babies born in the U.S. in a given year prevents 14 million infections and saves 33,000 lives. Savings reach $10 billion in medical costs by the time the children reach adolescence.

Do vaccines cause autism?
The best scientific evidence says no. Experts are instead focusing on genetic and environmental factors.

Will my child react badly to immunization?
The vast majority will not. Genetic-screening advances may help doctors identify the few who might.

Is mercury still used in vaccines?
Only in the flu vaccine. By 2001 new formulations of vaccines were introduced, which dramatically cut mercury exposure for 6-month-olds. The new vaccines had no discernible effect on autism rates.

Must I vaccinate my children?
Yes. All but two states allow exemptions if families object to vaccines on religious grounds; 20 allow them to opt out for philosophical reasons.

■ On the Horizon Briefs

Squeaky Clean
Even as fears of superbugs grow, fewer of us are cleaning up

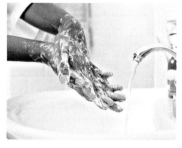

Hygiene is important, especially as bacteria become increasingly resistant to antibiotics. But fewer us are washing our hands after using public rest rooms, a 2007 study found. According to the survey, 77% of men and women said they washed their hands after using a public rest room. The results reflected a steep fall-off from 2005, when 84% of men and women said they washed their hands after using a public facility. As for gender differences, in 2007 some 88% of women claimed they washed up, vs. 66% of men, while in 2005, 90% of women said they did, vs. 75% of men. For those who do wash their hands, the National Institutes of Health recommends scrubbing briskly for 20 seconds.

Fighting Bird Flu A new vaccine is safer, more effective and faster to make

Since 1997, when bird flu first emerged in Hong Kong as a grave public-health menace, millions of birds have been culled in Asia, even as scientists have searched for a vaccine to protect humans against the virus. While a vaccine against the virus that causes this form of flu exists, it isn't as effective as doctors would like. But scientists writing in the *New England Journal of Medicine* in June 2008 declared they had succeeded in developing a whole-virus vaccine that appears to be safer and more effective, and, perhaps more importantly, can be manufactured much more quickly than conventional vaccines. The key to the new approach: using cells, rather than eggs, to culture the flu viruses that end up in the vaccine.

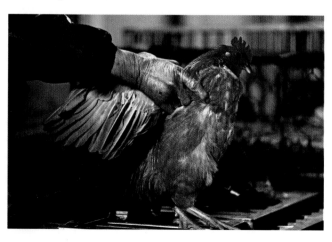

School Bug A tough breed of staph hits our classrooms

Many U.S. schools are scrubbing their hallways, gyms and locker rooms with extra care these days, alarmed by the threat of a potent bacteria, methicillin-resistant *Staphylococcus aureus* (MRSA). Efforts to fight the bug first ramped up in the fall of 2007, after three students contracted serious cases of the infection and died. The concern: like many of the new strains of bacterial superbugs, MRSA has developed resistance to penicillin and other standard antibiotics.

Since the 1960s, hospitals have been battling the bug among their patients; the concern now is that more and more cases seem to be coming from other than health-care settings. Indeed, health officials class the infection as two types: hospital-associated MRSA, which generally afflicts health-care professionals, and community-associated

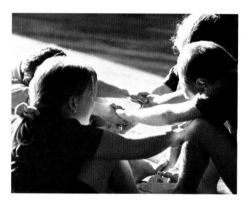

MRSA, which strikes schools, community centers, sports locker rooms and other locales where skin-to-skin contact is frequent. Most cases of MRSA are mild, appearing as red bumps on the skin. It's the less common, more serious MRSA infections that pose a serious threat; they can enter the bloodstream and damage essential tissues.

Teachers, parents and coaches seeking to keep the bug at bay should follow a few simple rules. Schools, locker rooms and health clubs should be kept clean. Parents and children should stay alert to news of outbreaks. And everyone should take care to keep hands washed and cuts covered with bandages. Bacteria can't thrive where they aren't welcome.

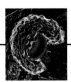

AIDS: Intractable
A new vaccine fails to stop the killer

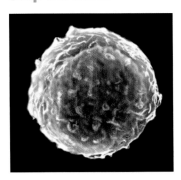

For more than 25 years, scientists have been trying to develop a vaccine against AIDS—and they continue to be disappointed. Many had high hopes for a novel strategy to protect the body against HIV, but in the fall of 2007 health officials declared that this vaccine too had failed.

In the new shot, scientists inserted three HIV genes into an ordinary cold virus and injected it into the body. Immune-system dendritic cells would, they hoped, gobble up the virus and then display its gene markers—along with those of HIV. This would teach the immune system's T cells (above) to recognize and kill AIDS-infected cells. But they did not, and the HIV virus once again foiled researchers' best attempts at controlling the infection.

The failure left the scientists wondering if a cold virus was the right carrier. Such viruses do a good job of ferrying HIV genes, but they are so common that most people have some tolerance to them, and thus the immune system waves them past without getting too excited by them. The next step: abandon the cold virus and switch to another one, perhaps chicken pox. AIDS is persistent, but the game is long—and science is patient.

Getting the Lead Out Americans tossed out millions of toys, but lead may be lurking in many homes

"Made in China" took on an ominous connotation in recent years as more than 20 million toys manufactured for companies like Mattel were recalled for unsafe levels of lead. The neurotoxin can accumulate in the body and cause ongoing learning and physical disabilities in children. While trace amounts are found in lipstick and candy—the FDA has set a limit of 0.1 parts per million—lead in paint and plastic used in toys is troublesome since children are more likely to ingest it while chewing and sucking on favorite playthings.

The best strategy for concerned parents is to remove any toy that manufacturers and government health officials have identified as containing lead. And if your children are playing with toys that have peeling or chipped paint, doctors recommend a blood test. The average lead level for children in the U.S. is 2 mcg/dL of blood. A level of 10 or higher is cause for concern.

And despite the fact that lead-tainted toys have received all the attention, it's worth remembering that the most common source of elevated lead in American children isn't toys; it's old paint chipping off the walls in houses built before 1978—that's when paint containing the metal was banned in the U.S.

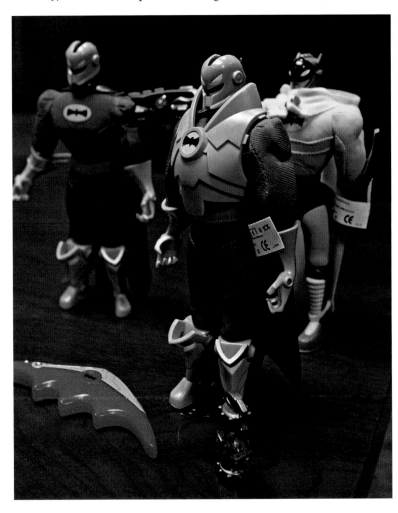